# SELF-INJURIOUS BEHAVIORS

## Assessment and Treatment

# CLINICAL

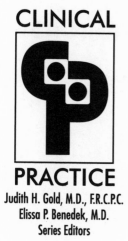

# PRACTICE

Judith H. Gold, M.D., F.R.C.P.C.
Elissa P. Benedek, M.D.
Series Editors

# SELF-INJURIOUS BEHAVIORS

## Assessment and Treatment

*Edited by*

Daphne Simeon, M.D.

Eric Hollander, M.D.

American Psychiatric Publishing, Inc.

Washington, DC
London, England

**Note:** The authors have worked to ensure that all information in this book concerning drug dosages, schedules, and routes of administration is accurate as of the time of publication and consistent with standards set by the U.S. Food and Drug Administration and the general medical community. As medical research and practice advance, however, therapeutic standards may change. For this reason and because human and mechanical errors sometimes occur, we recommend that readers follow the advice of a physician who is directly involved in their care or the care of a member of their family.

Copyright © 2001 American Psychiatric Publishing, Inc.
ALL RIGHTS RESERVED
Manufactured in the United States of America on acid-free paper

04   03   02        4   3   2
First Edition

American Psychiatric Publishing, Inc.
1400 K Street, N.W.
Washington, DC 20005
www.appi.org

**Library of Congress Cataloging-in-Publication Data**
Self-injurious behaviors : assessment and treatment / edited by Daphne Simeon, Eric Hollander.
    p. cm.
  Includes bibliographical references and index.
  ISBN 0-88048-808-5 (alk. paper)
    1. Self-injurious behavior. 2. Self-mutilation. 3. Psychology, Pathological. I. Simeon, Daphne. II. Hollander, Eric, 1957-

RC569.5.S48 S454 2001
616.85'82--dc21

                                                        00-061807

**British Library Cataloguing in Publication Data**
A CIP record is available from the British Library.

Cover photo: Copyright© Digital Vision® Ltd. All rights reserved.

12-15-05

# Contents

# Contributors

**Bonnie Aronowitz, Ph.D.**
Assistant Professor, Department of Psychiatry, Mount Sinai School of Medicine, New York, New York

**Milton Brown, M.A.**
Graduate student, Department of Psychology, University of Washington, Seattle, Washington

**Armando R. Favazza, M.D.**
Professor, Department of Psychiatry, University of Missouri—Columbia School of Medicine, Columbia, Missouri

**Robert Grossman, M.D.**
Assistant Professor; Director, Mount Sinai Integrated Treatment Program for Personality Disorders; and Medical Director, Mount Sinai Specialized Treatment Program for Holocaust Survivors, Department of Psychiatry, Mount Sinai School of Medicine, New York, New York

**Orna Guralnik, Psych.D.**
Assistant Research Professor, Department of Psychiatry, Mount Sinai School of Medicine, New York, New York

**Eric Hollander, M.D.**
Professor; Director of Clinical Psychopharmacology; Director, Compulsive, Impulsive, and Anxiety Disorders Program; and Clinical Director, Seaver Autism Research Center, Department of Psychiatry, Mount Sinai School of Medicine, New York, New York

**Andre Ivanoff, Ph.D.**
Associate Professor, School of Social Work, Columbia University, New York, New York

**Marsha M. Linehan, Ph.D.**
Professor and Director, Behavioral Research and Therapy Clinic, Department of Psychology, University of Washington, Seattle, Washington

**Dana J. H. Niehaus, M.B.**
Director, Psychiatric Genetics Program, Department of Psychiatry, University of Stellenbosch, Cape Town, South Africa

**Larry Siever, M.D.**
Professor; Director, Mount Sinai Mood and Personality Disorders Research Program; Director, Mount Sinai Outpatient Department; and Director, BVA Mental Illness Research, Education and Clinical Center (MIRECC), Department of Psychiatry, Mount Sinai School of Medicine, New York, New York

**Daphne Simeon, M.D.**
Assistant Professor and Director, Medical Student Education, Department of Psychiatry, Mount Sinai School of Medicine, New York, New York

**Dan J. Stein, M.B.**
Director, MRC Research Unit on Anxiety Disorders, and Director of Research, Department of Psychiatry, University of Stellenbosch, Cape Town, South Africa

# Introduction

## to the Clinical Practice Series

*T*he Clinical Practice Series is dedicated to the support of continuing education and enrichment for the practicing clinician. Books in this series address topics of concern and importance to psychiatrists and other mental health clinicians. Each volume provides up-to-date literature reviews and emphasizes the most recent treatment approaches to psychiatric illnesses. Theoretical and scientific data are applied to clinical situations, and case illustrations are used extensively to increase the relevance of the material for the practitioner.

Each year the series publishes a number of books dealing with all aspects of clinical practice. From time to time some of these publications may be revised and updated. Some books in the series are written by a single clinician widely acknowledged to be an authority on the topic area; other series books are edited volumes in which knowledgeable practitioners contribute chapters in their areas of expertise. Still other series books have their origins in presentations for an American Psychiatric Association Annual Meeting. All contain the newest research and clinical information available on the subjects discussed.

The Clinical Practice Series provides enrichment reading in a compact format specially designed to meet the continuing-education needs of the busy mental health clinician.

Judith H. Gold, C.M., M.D., F.R.C.P.C., F.R.A.N.Z.C.P.
*Series Editor*

# Introduction

*P*eople can inflict direct and intentional physical injury on themselves without an intent to die in many different ways, some culturally sanctioned and others pathologic. The latter self-injurious behaviors (SIBs) make up the subject of this book. The phenomenon of people physically hurting themselves is heterogeneous in its nature, disturbing in its impact on the self and on others, frightening in its blatant maladaptiveness, and often indicative of serious developmental disturbances, breaks with reality, or deficits in the regulation of affects, aggressive impulses, or self states. All of these factors can at times impede clinicians from understanding, addressing, and treating self-injury in a thorough and confident fashion. Further complexity is added by the large and diverse scope of psychiatric conditions in which these behaviors are encountered, such as pervasive developmental disorders, Tourette's syndrome, mental retardation, psychosis, impulse control disorders, stereotypic movement disorders, and severe personality disorders, to name some common ones. A distinct descriptive nosologic classification of these behaviors, which would encompass their major phenomenologic presentations, has been proposed by several authors who have worked in this field. Research into the biologic underpinnings of SIBs is still in its infancy, and therefore the question of unifying neurochemical processes or circuitry that may underlie these diverse behaviors remains unanswered.

In this book we present the entire scope of SIBs, classifying them into four broad categories: stereotypic, major, compulsive, and impulsive. Stereotypic SIB is seen mostly by clinicians working with the developmentally disabled, and major SIB is an unusual complication of psychosis that a clinician might only rarely encounter but is unlikely to forget. Compulsive and impulsive SIB are far more commonly encountered by most clinicians and are therefore given greater emphasis in this volume. An introductory chapter presents a description of the breadth of SIBs, proposes a classification system, and offers general guidelines to the evaluation of SIB. Specific chapters follow for each category of SIB on phenomenology, biologic and psychologic theories, and treatment approaches, both pharmacologic and psychotherapeutic. In writing this book for clinicians, we have aimed to make it sophisticated in its data base and research findings and thorough in its referencing, yet succinct and closely tied to clinical material and therapeutic interventions so as to be readily applicable to thinking about and working with self-injuring patients.

Daphne Simeon, M.D.
Eric Hollander, M.D.

# CHAPTER 1

# Self-Injurious Behaviors
## Phenomenology and Assessment

Daphne Simeon, M.D.
Armando R. Favazza, M.D.

## Self-Injurious Behaviors: How to Define Them?

Self-injurious behaviors (SIBs) are multiple and diverse in their presentation and often bewildering and vexing in the powers that drive them, their frequently blatant self-destructiveness, and the call for effective intervention. Various terms have been used over the years to name behaviors centering around intentional but nonsuicidal physical injury to the self that variably reflect descriptive aspects or assumptions about intent and are sometimes derogatory and moralistically tinged. Some of the more common terms include *partial suicide* (Menninger 1935, 1938), *antisuicide* (Simpson 1976), *deliberate self-harm* (Pattison and Kahan 1983), *delicate self-cutting* (Pao 1969), *wrist-cutting syndrome* (Graff and Mallin 1967; R.J. Rosenthal et al. 1972), and of course the ubiquitous term *self-mutilation*. We prefer to use the term *self-injurious behaviors* in this book because it is purely descriptive, suggests that a diversity of such behaviors exists, makes no allusion to motivation, and is not sensationalistic or derogatory.

We define SIBs as all behaviors involving the deliberate infliction of direct physical harm to one's own body without any intent to die as a consequence of the behavior. In this definition, the term *deliberate* implies conscious intent rather than unconsciously driven motivation; accident-prone individuals, for example, may have an unconscious need to be injured or to injure themselves but do not do it "deliberately." On the other hand, an individual who self-injures during a dissociative episode may have no memory of performing the behavior but may have had conscious intent to self-injure while in an altered state. "Direct" physical harm implies injury that is pretty much immediate in impact; liver damage caused by alcohol or lung destruction caused by cigarette smoking would not be included here, even if known to the subject. The physical injury may be external, such as skin cutting or picking, or internal, such as the ingestion of sharp objects commonly found in prison populations. _Without any intent to die_ implies just that, because the intensity and seriousness of suicidal intent can be variable and ambivalence is commonly encountered. Asked if they wished to die as a result of the particular act, patients who engage in self-injury are able to answer "no." On the other hand, individuals who self-injure can often feel very dysphoric, depressed, or desperate when they hurt themselves and may be experiencing suicidal ideation. They are still able to describe, however, that their SIB itself had no suicidal intent; although often an expression of how bad they were feeling at the time, the behavior in itself it is not intended to kill and may even bring relief.

## Classification of Self-Injurious Behaviors

Based then on the above descriptive definition, how can we go about classifying the bewildering variety of SIBs that we may encounter in our clinical practice? To this day, general clinicians and research experts in the field have not agreed on which behaviors to include under the rubric of self-injury or on how to then proceed and categorize them into meaningful groups. A typical example of this dilemma is trichotillomania—some would not classify it in the broad schema of SIBs (Winchel and Stanley 1991). We have chosen to include it under this category because pulling one's own hair does inflict bodily injury in the broadest sense, although patients will most commonly deny that this is the intent of the behavior. SIBs are largely underrepresented in our current classification system; the DSM-IV (American Psychiatric Association 1994) offers few and inconsistent guidelines in this regard. The limited research on SIBs has probably delayed their emergence as distinct nosologic entities that may warrant their own classification. They are commonly viewed as symptoms within the context of a particular psychiatric disorder (e.g., schizophrenia, autism, borderline personality), and it remains an open question whether SIBs across diagnostic categories share common features in phenomenology, biologic underpinnings, or treatment responses that might justify distinct classification.

DSM-IV offers four rather disparate diagnoses under which many but not all SIBs can be "fitted":

1. Trichotillomania, under the Axis I Impulse-Control Disorders Not Elsewhere Classified. This classification emphasizes the increasing tension immediately prior to, and the gratification or relief during, the recurrent hair-pulling behavior.
2. Impulse-Control Disorder Not Otherwise Specified. SIBs are not explicitly mentioned in this category but may certainly be classified here if, as with trichotillomania above, they fit the impulse dyscontrol criteria regarding irresistible urge and subsequent relief.
3. Axis II Borderline Personality Disorder. One of the nine diagnostic criteria for this classification is "recurrent suicidal behavior, gestures, or threats, or self-mutilating behavior" (American Psychiatric Association 1994, p. 654)
4. Stereotypic Movement Disorder with Self-Injurious Behavior, under Other Disorders of Infancy, Childhood, or Adolescence. This disorder comprises behaviors that are "repetitive, often seemingly driven, and nonfunctional" (American Psychiatric Association 1994, p. 118). Examples mentioned include head banging, self-biting, skin picking, or hitting parts of one's body. Mental retardation may or may not be present, and the behavior should not be accounted for by a pervasive developmental disorder such as autism, by obsessive-compulsive disorder (OCD), or by trichotillomania.

Reviewing the heterogeneous classification options above, which include disorders of childhood or adulthood, Axis I or Axis II, and disorder-based or behavior-based, it becomes readily apparent that they contain an element of arbitrariness and raise numerous questions and dilemmas regarding classification. For example, trichotillomania is excluded from Stereotypic Movement Disorders even though it fits the description and often commences before adulthood—seemingly it is excluded simply because it enjoys a diagnostic niche of its own. Furthermore, an assumption about etiology is made in some but not others of the above diagnoses, such as impulse control dysregulation in trichotillomania. However, this assumption may be problematic given the absence of urge and gratification in a significant minority of cases (Christenson et al. 1991a, 1991b), the absence of association with impulsive personality (Christenson et al. 1992), and the frequent comorbidity (Christenson 1991a) and shared characteristics (Stein et al. 1995) with OCD.

Would picking one's own skin, a behavior frequently comorbid with trichotillomania (Simeon et al. 1997a), similarly be classified under Stereotypic Movement Disorders or Impulse-Control Disorders Not Otherwise Specified? What criteria other than age would this decision be based on? A more repetitive and driven picture would support the former diagnosis, whereas an impulsive picture would support the latter—admittedly, these are distinctions that can be difficult to make and are again not free of assumptions about mechanisms or motivations. Would the classification change yet again if the skin-picking patient also carried the diagnosis of borderline personality disorder?

Another diagnostic dilemma is the unique link implied between self-mutilation and borderline personality disorder to the exclusion of other personality disorders that can involve such behavior, albeit less often (Simeon et al. 1992). Finally, psychotic acts of self-injury, often major and dramatic such as castration or eye enucleation, are difficult to classify in the above schema.

Over the past decade, Favazza has proposed the most widely used system for classifying SIBs, initially in collaboration with Rosenthal (Favazza and Rosenthal 1990) and more recently expanded in work with Simeon (Favazza and Simeon 1995). Four large categories are proposed based on this schema that encompass the entire spectrum of SIBs (Table 1–1). Although purely phenomenologically based and therefore simplistic, this schema offers significant advantages, such as its comprehensiveness and its clinical usefulness (Favazza 1998). Each category of self-injury tends to be more prevalent in certain mental disorders. This schema largely disregards etiology and is subject to future modifications as more extensive research in self-injury unfolds, especially in the area of biologic determinants. We propose four major categories of SIB: 1) stereotypic, 2) major, 3) compulsive, and 4) impulsive. Each is presented in a summary description in this chapter. The remainder of this book is organized into sections according to this classification, addressing the biology, psychology, and treatment approaches to each of the four categories of self-injury. We end this chapter with guidelines for psychiatric interviewing, systematic assessment, and determination of severity and change of SIBs.

## Spanning the Normal to the Abnormal: Self-Injury in Culture and Religion

In his book *Bodies Under Siege: Self-Mutilation and Body Modification in Culture and Psychiatry*, Favazza (1996), tracing from prehistoric times to the

**Table 1–1.** Classification of self-injurious behaviors

| Category | Behaviors | Tissue damage | Rate | Pattern | Disorders |
|---|---|---|---|---|---|
| Stereotypic | Head banging<br>Self-hitting<br>Lip or hand chewing<br>Skin picking or scratching<br>Self-biting<br>Hair pulling | Mild to severe (even life threatening) | Highly repetitive<br>Fixed | Fixed<br>Contentless<br>Driven | Mental retardation<br>Autism<br>Lesch-Nyhan<br>Cornelia de Lange<br>Prader-Willi |
| Major | Castration<br>Eye enucleation<br>Limb amputation | Severe or life threatening | Isolated | Impulsive or planned<br>Concrete symbolism | Psychosis (schizophrenia, affective, organic)<br>Intoxications<br>Severe character disorders<br>Transsexualism |
| Compulsive | Hair pulling<br>Skin picking<br>Nail biting | Mild to moderate | Repetitive | Compulsive (with impulsive traits)<br>Ritualized<br>Sometimes symbolic | Trichotillomania<br>Stereotypic movement disorder with self-injurious behavior |
| Impulsive | Skin cutting<br>Skin burning<br>Self-hitting | Mild to moderate | Isolated or habitual, not highly repetitive | Impulsive (may have compulsive traits)<br>Ritualized<br>Often symbolic | Borderline/antisocial personality disorder<br>Other impulsive personality disorders<br>Abuse/trauma/dissociation/posttraumatic stress disorder<br>Eating disorders |

present, extensively researched and vividly described various forms of "culturally sanctioned self-mutilative rituals and practices." We very briefly summarize these here. *Cultural rituals* are ritualized activities repeated over many generations of a particular culture, woven into the society's fabric of traditions and beliefs, and shared by many of its members. For example, in the Sun Dance of the Plains Indians, selected young men struggle until skewers inserted under the muscles of their chest and back break free. *Cultural practices*, on the other hand, are activities with little symbolic significance in the culture, such as ear piercing in our own.

Culturally ritualized self-injury may promote three broad societal goals, as described by Favazza (1996): healing, spirituality, and order. Healing rituals that involve self-mutilation are widespread in the world: Muslim healers in Morocco slash open their heads so that the sick may eat bread dipped in the blood to get well. In New Guinea, men mimic women's menstrual cycle in pursuit of health and purification by periodically inducing nasal hemorrhages. In South Africa, holes were made in skulls in order to relieve headaches by allowing the evil spirits to escape. Spiritual ends include attainment of higher spiritual states and appeasing deitites or spirits. For example, the Eastern Orthodox Skiptsi sect engaged in self-castration to avoid temptation into sin and to recapture the purity before the original sin. Aztecs and Mayans anointed sacred idols with blood from their penises to show penitence and devotion. Self-mutitative practices aimed at attaining, maintaining, or proclaiming social status and order are also widespread. African tribes may cut off specific fingers to indicate their clan. The Flathead Indians molded the skulls of their children to achieve a specific shape. Adolescent self-mutilating rituals may herald initiation into adulthood and can include skin, nasal, and penile piercing and cutting.

In contrast with culturally sanctioned self-mutilation, pathologic self-mutilation tends to be viewed negatively by the general culture, lacks culturally shared meanings although it may be rich in individual meanings and symbolisms, and is not practiced by large sections of a society. Pathologic SIBs are described below.

## Stereotypic Self-Injurious Behaviors

*Stereotypic SIBs* refers to highly repetitive, monotonous, fixed, often rhythmic, seemingly highly driven, and usually contentless (i.e., devoid of thought, affect, and meaning) acts, which can widely range in self-inflicted tissue injury from mild to severe or even life-threatening at times. They are more likely not to occur in private compared with the other three categories of SIB, are commonly but not necessarily associated with some degree of mental retardation, and appear more strongly driven by biology than are other types of SIB. Common conditions associated with stereotypic SIB include mental retardation, autism, and syndromes such as Lesch-Nyhan, Cornelia de Lange, and Prader-Willi. We present here a brief description of such behaviors, whose neurobiology and treatment is extensively described in Chapter 2.

SIB is quite common in individuals with mental retardation; estimates range from 3% to 46% (Bodfish et al. 1995; Winchel and Stanley 1991). In a very large survey of 10,000 mentally retarded state school residents, 14% exhibited SIB such as head banging, head and body hitting, self-biting, severe scratching or hair pulling, and eye or throat gouging (Griffin et al. 1986). Both institutionalization, especially in environments that do not offer optimal stimulation, and the severity of mental retardation tend to correlate with the presence and severity of SIB (King 1993; Winchel and Stanley 1991).

Various syndromes may exhibit SIB, and we describe here a few in which SIB is a central feature. Lesch-Nyhan syndrome is a rare X-linked recessive disorder of purine synthesis found only in boys. Patients present with various neuropsychiatric symptoms, including spasticity, dystonia, choreoathetosis, mental retardation, aggression, and SIB. These unfortunate children profoundly self-mutilate their bodies if they are not kept in restraints. Typical behaviors are biting and chewing off lips, tongue, and fingers, although other behaviors such as head banging, eye poking, and self-scratching also occur. Onset of SIB may be as early as in infancy or as late as in adolescence (Jankovic 1988; Lesch and Nyhan 1964; Shear et al. 1971).

Cornelia de Lange syndrome is a rare congenital disorder characterized by severe mental retardation, a distinctive appearance, and SIB in about half of of the children with the disorder. SIBs include lip biting, self-scratching, head and face slapping, and excessive grooming behaviors such as hand licking and hair stroking (Bryson et al. 1971; Singh and Pulman 1979).

Prader-Willi syndrome is a congenital disorder and comprises one of the five most common birth defects (Prader et al. 1956). It is characterized by hyperphagia and obesity, hypogonadism, mental retardation, and behavioral disturbances that include temper outbursts, self-injury, and obsessive-compulsive symptoms (D.J. Clarke et al. 1989; Stein et al. 1994). SIBs include skin and nose picking, nail biting, and hair pulling; skin picking has been described as the "best cutaneous symptom in the recognition of Prader-Willi syndrome" (Schepis et al. 1994, p. 866). SIBs are common and do not necessarily correlate with cognitive impairment (Stein et al. 1994).

Autism is a pervasive developmental disorder characterized by social deficits and restrictive stereotyped behaviors. Stereotyped SIBs are common in autism and may include hand biting, self-scratching, head banging, self-hitting or -pinching, and hair pulling (Rothenberger 1993); these may often be among the most troubling manifestations of the condition, requiring behavioral and/or pharmacologic management.

## Major Self-Injurious Behaviors

*Major SIBs*, as the term suggests, encompass the most dramatic and often life-threatening forms of self-injury and involve major and often irreversible destruction of body tissue. They most commonly occur as isolated rather than repetitive events. Castration, eye enucleation, and (to a lesser degree) amputation of extremities are the most common of these behaviors. They may be carefully planned out or highly impulsive in nature and are by far more common in psychotic states. Schizophrenia is the most common disorder in which major SIB is encountered, but other conditions, more often but not exclusively psychotic, have been reported in association with major SIB including intoxications (Moskovitz and Byrd 1983; R.J. Rosenthal et al. 1972), encephalitis (Goodhart and Savitsky 1933), congential sensory neuropathy (Dubovsky 1978), depression or mania (Martin and Gattaz 1991; Thompson and Abraham 1983), severe character disorders (Nakaya 1996), and transsexualism (Krieger et al. 1982).

Genital SIB may be the most common type in this category and appears to be at least 10 times as common in men as in women, although exact numbers are unreliable given the largely retrospective compilation of cases and series on which our knowledge is based (Greilsheimer and Groves 1979). Self-inflicted injuries include complete or partial transection of the penis, removal of the testicles, or both. The large majority of these individuals appear to suffer from a schizophrenic or affective psychosis (Martin and Gattaz 1991).

With psychosis, major SIB typically occurs within the context of delusions and/or command hallucinations; the most common themes of these center around sexual temptation, sin, self-punishment, and salvation (R.A. Clark 1981; DeMuth et al. 1983). Religious delusions are quite common (Nakaya 1996). Acting on these psychotic beliefs is further facilitated by the concrete thinking that is typically characteristic of schizophrenic patients (e.g., that the genitals are the cause of the evil and their removal will lead to redemption) combined with poor impulse control and, interestingly, a very heightened pain threshold in these states so that many patients report having experienced little or no pain during these acts (Bach-Y-Rita 1974).

The other most common form of major SIB, ocular SIB, occurs mostly in psychotic individuals with sexual and/or religious themes (very much like genital SIB) as well as in depressions or intoxications (Kennedy and Feldman 1994). It again occurs more commonly in men, for reasons that are unknown but could possibly be related to the generally greater association of highly violent outwardly or self-directed acts with male gender. SIBs may involve complete removal of the eye, cutting, puncturing, or blinding with caustic agents.

Acts of major SIB typically constitute psychiatric as well as medical emergencies and involve salvaging the injured part, if possible, and understanding, treating, and preventing the recurrence of similar precipitating states. Chapter 3 addresses in detail the presentations, underpinnings, precipitants, and therapeutic interventions for major SIB.

## Compulsive Self-Injurious Behaviors

In this section we include repetitive, often ritualistic behaviors that typically occur multiple times per day, such as trichotillomania (hair pulling), onychophagia (nail biting), and skin picking or skin scratching (neurotic excoriations). Of these, trichotillomania is by far the more extensively investigated and the only one diagnostically classified as a discrete disorder in the DSM-IV. It is categorized as an impulse control disorder—that is, conceptualized primarily as a behavior occurring in response to an irresistible urge and resulting in gratification. Indeed, clinical studies show that most patients with trichotillomania do report mounting tension and relief associated with the behavior, but a minority of patients report neither (Christenson et al. 1991a). Patients may also describe the behavior as occurring automatically, without any conscious urge, or with a complex variety of associated thoughts and affects (Christenson et al. 1993). In a survey of individuals with trichotillomania, factor analysis revealed six motivational clusters underlying the behavior (Simeon et al. 1997c).

Often, hair pulling may be experienced as quite dystonic and intrusive as opposed to a pleasurable urge; patients may feel compelled to execute it but may wish to resist it with variable success. Increasing anxiety with subsequent tension relief is commonly described. In this respect the behavior is phenomenologically reminiscent of the compulsions found in patients with OCD who have few or no obsessions; it has been described as an OCD-related disorder (Stein et al. 1995; Swedo 1993). In one series of patients with trichotillomania, 15% had a history of lifetime OCD, and an additional 18% had a history of obsessive-compulsive symptoms (Christenson et al. 1991a). These rates are at least five times higher than those found in the general population. Indeed, rating scales devised by various investigators for quantifying the severity of trichotillomania and its response to treatment are patterned after and measure similar aspects as scales of OCD (Swedo et al. 1989b; Winchel et al. 1992). Some researchers have proposed a neuroethologic model to explain compulsive self-injury such as hair pulling as well as OCD compulsions such as washing, postulating that these compulsions are dysregulated, excessive, and repetitive versions of normal adaptive grooming behaviors (Swedo and Rapoport 1991). Given the highly repetitive nature of the behavior, with its compulsive features and similarities to OCD as opposed to the vividly more impulsive nature of SIBs such as skin cutting described later in this chapter, we have chosen to classify hair pulling and other similar behaviors under the rubric of compulsive SIB. At the same time, we recognize that this is probably an oversimplification and that these behaviors are best described as having both compulsive and impulsive features (Stein et al. 1995) but fall more at the compulsive end of the impulsivity-compulsivity spectrum. The fourth SIB category, impulsive SIB, also has both impulsive and compulsive features but falls more at the impulsive end of the spectrum.

Compulsive SIBs other than hair pulling, such as skin picking and nail biting, appear to be quite common yet have received much less attention in the psychiatric literature. The relative absence of epidemiologic or clinical studies examining the lifetime prevalence and temporal patterns of overlap or symptom substitution among various SIBs seriously limits our knowledge in this very interesting arena. Additionally, a challenging area of study is the comorbidity and relationship between compulsive and impulsive SIBs. Although it had serious methodologic limitations given survey sampling, one study of subjects with trichotillomania (Simeon et al. 1997a) found considerable lifetime comorbidity of compulsive and impulsive SIBs, with rates of 31% for nail biting, 28% for skin picking, 14% for skin scratching, 10% for skin cutting, 10% for self-hitting, 7% for self-biting, 7% for head banging, and below 5% for miscellaneous SIBs. Not surprisingly, impulsive SIB was more episodic, whereas compulsive SIB occurred with greater frequency, and more than half of the group engaged in multiple self-injury. In a group of 60 hair-pulling subjects interviewed, *impulsive* comorbid behaviors included self-cutting in 5%, self-burning in 3%, and self-hitting in 3%, whereas more *compulsive* behaviors such as picking, biting, and chewing co-occurred in 85% (Christenson et al. 1991a). Conversely, in a large sample of women with impulsive SIB who were surveyed by questionnaire, 10% engaged in hair pulling (Favazza and Conterio 1989). Indeed, in a study of patients with bulimia, both impulsive and compulsive SIBs were examined and on analysis were found to separate into two factors (Favaro and Santonastaso 1998). In addition to skin cutting and skin burning, the impulsive factor included other impulsive behaviors such as suicide attempts, substance abuse, and laxative abuse, whereas the compulsive factor comprised hair pulling, nail biting, and self-induced vomiting, thus supporting the classification proposed herein by Favazza and Simeon (1995).

In the following section we describe some of the most commonly encountered compulsive SIBs, the neurobiology, pharmacotherapy, and psychotherapy of which are outlined in detail in Chapters 4 and 5.

## Trichotillomania

Trichotillomania consists of abnormal, repetitive hair pulling, and any body hair may be targeted. Pulling may be confined to a single site, but most patients pull hair from multiple sites. Trichotillomania either appears, undergoes acute exacerbation, or resurfaces during periods of heightened stress or anxiety but may also occur during periods of inactivity and relaxation (Stanley et al. 1992), boredom, or in response to other specific cues such as negative affective states (Christenson et al. 1993). Scalp hairs are most commonly pulled, but other common sites of hair pulling include the eyebrows, eyelashes, beard, axillae, extremities, and pubic area (Christenson et al. 1991a). Individuals with trichotillomania are often secretive about their behavior and many conceal hair pulling and the consequent thinning or bald patches by using wigs, scarves, or strategic hairstyles for the scalp, make-up for eyelashes and eyebrows, or even new cosmetic tattooing techniques for eyebrow replacement. Because of the secretive nature of the disorder and the associated feelings of shame and low self-esteem, many individuals do not seek treatment for a long time. Trichotillomania can cause marked distress, may significantly interfere with daily activities, may lead to a markedly restricted lifestyle, and in extreme cases may ultimately result in complete social isolation.

Although no surveys of trichotillomania have been performed in the general population, more than 8 million individuals in the United States have been estimated to have the disorder (Azrin and Nunn 1973; Swedo et al. 1989a). Prevalence of hair pulling in adults is reported to be as high as 10%, but more severe cases accompanied by alopecia and marked distress are reported to affect approximately 1%–2% (Christenson et al. 1991b; Rothbaum et al. 1993). Age of onset of trichotillomania is generally in childhood or adolescence (Cohen et al. 1995).

Children and adults have extremely similar symptoms (Swedo et al. 1989b), but the number of children affected with trichotillomania has been estimated as seven times higher than that for adults. Moreover, trichotil-lomania in children has been reported to frequently co-occur with nail bit-ing, thumb sucking, nose picking, masturbation, poor peer relationships, and academic difficulties (Krishnan et al. 1985). Unlike the chronic, debil-itating trichotillomania of adolescence and young adulthood, early onset trichotillomania is usually reported to be benign and self-limiting (Stroud 1983) and usually does not continue into adolescence or adulthood (Oran-je et al. 1986). Some authors report no gender differences in trichotillo-mania, but most reports find women to be overrepresented in adult or adolescent clinical samples (Swedo et al. 1989b). The disorder may be more prevalent in boys in the preschool age group.

The self-injurious nature of the behavior is attested to by the local tis-sue irritation commonly observed in trichotillomania; multiple hairs are repetitively pulled from the same sites, and fingernails or tweezers are sometimes used to scratch the skin surface and remove short or impacted hairs. Patients often prolong their disfigurement by continuing to pull at the regrowing hair of bald spots. Trichotillomania may be accompanied by trichophagia, the mouthing or ingestion of the hair or its root. Physical complications may result such as gastrointestinal distress or bowel ob-struction caused by hairballs forming in the stomach (Reti-Gyorgy et al. 1997). Psychologic repercussions include negative self-image, low self-esteem, guilt, shame, and feelings of loss of control and depression as well as possible social isolation. Factors that predict self-esteem difficulties in female hair pullers are levels of depression and anxiety, frequency of hair pulling, and body dissatisfaction unrelated to hair pulling (Soriano et al. 1996). Depressive, anxiety (including OCD), and substance use disorders are frequently comorbid with trichotillomania (Swedo 1993; Winchel 1992). In their study of 60 adult hair-pulling subjects, Christenson et al. (1991a) found a lifetime prevalence of 56% for mood disorders, 57% for anxiety disorders, 22% for substance abuse, and 15% for OCD.

## Compulsive Skin Picking

Individuals who engage in compulsive skin picking frequently present to dermatologists, and it has been estimated that about 2% of dermatology clinic patients may suffer from this condition (Doran et al. 1985; Gupta et al. 1986). Prevalence in the general population or in psychiatric clinics is unknown. Skin picking is often not a transient behavior but may persist with a waxing and waning course over a lifetime. It should be viewed as pathologic when it becomes habitual, chronic, and extensive, leading to significant distress, dysfunction, or disfigurement.

Scant information is available on this condition in the psychiatric literature; however, two recent psychiatric studies have more extensively and systematically characterized larger samples of adult patients with skin picking (Arnold et al. 1998; Simeon et al. 1997b). The findings of these studies are fairly consistent and are summarized here. In both studies, most patients were women and their condition was chronic with a mean duration of one to two decades. In the first series (Simeon et al. 1997b), onset was at a notably younger age than in the second series (Arnold et al. 1998)—16 versus 38 years of age, respectively. The most common comorbidities in both series were with mood, anxiety, and substance use disorders. Single or multiple sites were excoriated. The face was the most common site in both studies; other common sites included the scalp, arms, back, and legs. Few individuals had underlying skin conditions such as acne or eczema, although most were picking at minimal perceived irregularities of "normal" skin and thus creating and perpetuating lesions. One study (Arnold et al. 1998) described various skin sensations, most commonly pruritus, preceding the behavior in most subjects, whereas in the other study (Simeon et al. 1997b) this was true in a minority of subjects. This difference might be explained by the largely dermatologic referral base in the former study. The average patient engaged in 12 episodes or 2.5 hours of skin picking daily, and all experienced distress over variably feeling ashamed, socially humiliatiated, out of control, hopeless, or self-destructive (Simeon et al. 1997b). Impairment commonly was related to withdrawal and restrictions imposed by the desire to hide scarred or disfigured body parts in social, occupational, and intimate settings or related to time management, loss of sleep, or latenesses secondary to the behavior. Both studies found, in comparable percentages, that most subjects experienced mounting tension before the act (79%–81%), relief after the act (52%–79%), or both (68%–90%). One study quantified this behavior as highly dystonic and moderately resisted but poorly controlled (Simeon et al. 1997b), whereas the other study found a modified obsessive-compulsive scale mean score of 16 out of a maximum of 40 (Arnold et al. 1998). An approximately 10% lifetime comorbidity with trichotillomania was found in both studies. Lifetime comorbidity between skin picking and OCD varied from 6% to 19%, comparable with the 15% comorbidity between trichotillomania and OCD (Christenson et al. 1991a). It should be noted that these descriptive findings are comparable with those described previously for hair pulling, and in our opinion suggest that skin picking can best be descriptively classified, like hair pulling, as a compulsive SIB with impulsive features.

## Compulsive Nail Biting

Nail biting (onychophagia) is a very common behavior but is not always benign (Hadley 1984). It is highly prevalent in all age groups (Ballinger 1970; Massler and Malone 1950) and appears to be somewhat more common in females than in males (Bakwin 1971). Its prevalence in childhood is about 50% (Birch 1955); it can start very early and peaks between 10 and 18 years of age (Wechsler 1931). It gradually decreases over the adult years with a reported prevalence of 23% in young men (Pennington 1945) and 5% in elderly men and women (Ballinger 1970). Interestingly, monozygotic twins have much higher concordance for nail biting than dizygotic twins (Bakwin 1971).

Onychophagia should be viewed as pathologic when it is habitual, chronic, and extensive. It can result in various medical and dental complications such as serious infections, craniomandibular dysfunction, and orthodontic problems in addition to permanent nailbed damage and disfigurement of the nails and fingers. Onychotillomania, compulsive picking or tearing at the nails, is a variant of onychophagia. The very high prevalence of benign nail biting should not induce clinicians to prematurely dismiss this behavior before evaluating it fully and openly. In a more recent psychiatric treatment study that systematically assessed various characteristics of the participating 25 nail-biting adults, several characteristics comparable with those previously described for hair pulling and skin picking were described (Leonard et al. 1991). Women were predominant, and subjects had had the condition for at least two decades. Pain, disfigurement, and functional impairment were common, including difficulties using the hands or walking. Mood, anxiety, and substance use were common comorbid disorders; the prevalence of OCD could not be assessed because all subjects with histories of OCD were excluded. A small minority had Axis II personality disorders. It would be of great interest to conduct a large, systematic series that compares patients with hair pulling, skin picking, nail biting, or combinations of these behaviors using uniform recruitment methods, interviews, and questionnaires.

## Tourette's Disorder

Tourette's disorder (better known as Tourette's syndrome) is characterized by multiple motor and vocal tics with typical onset in early childhood. Compulsive SIBs are not uncommon in these individuals; prevalence ranges from 13% to 53% (Robertson 1989; Robertson et al. 1989). A wide range of behaviors may be seen, most commonly head banging, self-punching or -slapping, lip and tongue biting, eye poking, and skin picking. Serious medical complications have been described in these patients.

Self-injury appears not to correlate with intellectual function but rather with tic severity and with higher aggression and obsessionality (Robertson et al. 1989). Although Tourette's disorder and OCD show many similarities, SIB has been described as one differentiating characteristic between the two—one study demonstrated SIB prevalence of 50% in the former versus 12% in the latter (Pitman et al. 1987). Self-injury can add significant pain, impairment, and management challenges to these unfortunate patients who already suffer from disturbing tics.

## Impulsive Self-Injurious Behaviors

### General Description

Some individuals engage in impulsive SIBs only a limited number of times in their lifetimes, whereas others do so quite frequently and habitually. Favazza has proposed using the terms *episodic* and *repetitive* to differentiate these two types of patients (Favazza 1996; Favazza and Simeon 1995). In the repetitive type, self-injury may become an organizing and predominant preoccupation, with a seemingly addictive quality, that is incorporated into the individual's sense of identity. The self-injury may become almost an automatic response to various disturbing internal and external stimuli, typically beginning in adolescence and persisting for decades. Favazza and Simeon (1995) have proposed that repetitive impulsive self-injury be classified under "impulse control disorders not elsewhere classified" with the criteria described below.

The most common behaviors in the impulsive SIB category include skin cutting, skin burning, self-sticking with pins, and various ways of self-hitting using one's own body parts, objects, or by throwing oneself against objects. Although typically these behaviors can be conceptualized as acts of impulsive aggression, which justifies their inclusion in this category and is described in detail a little later, they are highly complex in their determinants, motivations, and precipitants. It can be generally said that these behaviors frequently permit those who engage in them to obtain rapid but short-lived relief from various intolerable states. In this sense, they serve a morbid and pathologic but life-sustaining function. A summary description follows.

1. Preoccupation with harming oneself physically
2. Recurrent failure to resist impulses to harm onself physically, resulting in the destruction or alteration of body tissue
3. Increasing sense of tension immediately prior to the act of self-injury

4. Gratification or sense of relief when committing the act of self-injury
5. No conscious suicidal intent associated with the act and it is not in response to psychosis, transexualism, mental retardation, or developmental disorder

As described in the compulsive self-injury section, the distinction between compulsive and impulsive repetitive self-injury may not always be sharp and clear. Impulsive repetitive self-injury can, at times, become so habitual as to occur on a daily or weekly basis and without clearly identifiable precipitating external events or affective states, as though it were a compulsion. It may be speculated that individuals who have an obsessive-compulsive predisposition may be more prone to become fixated on SIBs that were initially episodic and impulsive but over time became habitual and dystonic (Simeon et al. 1995). Interestingly, the few studies that have examined obsessionality in impulsive self-injury may indeed support such a notion. In one study comparing 22 female, inpatient, nonpsychotic "repetitive self-cutters" with 22 demographically matched inpatient control subjects, patients who engaged in self-injury were significantly more obsessional than control subjects but did not differ in depression, anxiety, phobia, or hysteria (A.R. Gardner and Gardner 1975). In another study comparing mutilating and nonmutilating antisocial women confined to a criminal ward, self-injuring subjects were found to be significantly more obsessional (McKerracher et al. 1968). It may therefore be that impulsive self-injury encompasses some obsessive-compulsive traits, just as compulsive self-injury may encompass some impulsive traits. Both types of traits could be postulated, each in their own way, to facilitate the perpetuation of the SIBs.

Although epidemiologic studies are lacking, it has been indirectly estimated that the incidence of impulsive self-injury may be at least 1 per 1,000 people annually (Favazza 1996). It is more common in females and typically begins in adolescence or early adulthood, although it has been described as early as the latency (Green 1978) or even the preschool (P.A. Rosenthal and Rosenthal 1984) years. It is more commonly associated with certain disorders, such as borderline personality disorder (D.L. Gardner and Cowdry 1985; Schaffer et al. 1982), antisocial personality disorder (Virkkunen 1976), posttraumatic stress disorder (Greenspan and Samuel 1989; Pitman 1990), dissociative disorders (Coons and Milstein 1990; Simeon et al. 1997c), and eating disorders (Favaro and Santonastaso 1998; Favazza et al. 1989; Garfinkel et al. 1980; Mitchell et al. 1986; Parkin and Eagles 1993). Of these diagnoses, the one that appears most commonly with SIB is borderline personality disorder; however, this is neither a necessary nor a sufficient condition, and the assumption of such could unfortunately lead to premature diagnostic formulation and closure.

Although the structure and context of the self-injury event can vary significantly from person to person, Liebenluft et al. (1987) outlined five descriptive stages that can be quite helpful in conceptualizing these behaviors. First is the precipitating event, often involving real or perceived loss, rejection, or abandonment. The second stage is the escalation of the intolerable affect, whether dysphoric or numb. Attempts to forestall self-injury (the third step) are followed by its execution (fourth), which is often accompanied by partial or total analgesia. The fifth and final stage is the aftermath, which commonly involves at least short-lived affective relief. Individuals describe various motivations or states that lead them to self-injure; these have been variably discussed and emphasized by numerous authors in both the descriptive and the psychodynamic literature (Favazza 1989, 1996; D.L. Gardner and Cowdry 1985; Graff and Mallin 1967; Kafka 1969; Leibenluft et al. 1987; Pao 1969). These states/motivations include releasing unbearable mounting tension; discharging rage directed at hated parts of the self, real or internalized others, or both; self-punishment; attempting to feel alive again by lifting depersonalization and emotional deadness; regaining a sense of control and omnipotence; self-soothing; reconfirming self boundaries; communicating with or controlling others; experiencing sexual excitement, euphoria, or titillation; relieving intolerable aloneness, alienation, hopelessness, or despair; combatting any desperate affects or thoughts; and expressing conflictual dissociative states. Naturally, some of these motivations overlap and the behavior can presumably serve multiple purposes in any particular individual; therefore, these complex states need to be sensitively attended to and understood.

The relationship between impulsive SIBs and suicide attempts warrants brief mention here. An act of wrist cutting, for example, should be viewed as self-mutilation only if indeed the patient describes no intent to die. Given that the wish to die is probably more often than not ambivalently held, the behavior would not be classified under self-injury if there was even some intent to die. On the other hand, the presence of suicidal ideation, either passive or active but not involving the particular behavior, does not exclude the diagnosis of self-injury, because people typically feel quite despairing or desperate when they self-injure and death is commonly on their minds. The incidence of suicidal ideation during self-mutilation has been found to vary from 28% to 41% (A.R. Gardner and Gardner 1975; Pattison and Kahan 1983). The coexistence of both behaviors in individuals with severe personality disorders may be more the rule than the exception. In a large, thoroughly studied series of chronically hospitalized, highly disturbed patients, of the 141 borderline females studied, 10 had histories of self-injury alone whereas 20 had histories of both self-injury and suicide attempts (Stone 1990). However, a 15-year follow-up of these patients suggested that history of self-injury alone was not a predictor of future suicide, whereas history of suicide attempts was; this observation indeed supports the distinct conceptualization of the two behaviors.

### Relationship to Impulsivity and Aggression

Descriptive and systematic data clearly reveal that these SIBs are typically impulsive, and hence their proposed classification in our schema. Bennum (1983) reported that 70% of self-mutilating individuals feel they have no control over the act. Favazza and Conterio (1989) reported that 78% of subjects in their sample decided to self-mutilate on the spur of the moment, and another 15% made the decision within 1 hour of the act. The act was then always (30%) or almost always (51%) carried out. In another sample, less than 15% of self-mutilating individuals reported any inner struggle to resist the behavior (A.R. Gardner and Gardner 1975). Simeon et al. (1992) found a significant correlation between the degree of self-mutilation and an independent measure of impulsivity.

With regard to aggression, studies of impulsive self-mutilators show that 18%–45% of individuals report anger toward themselves and 10%–32% report anger toward others leading up to the acts of self-injury (Bennum 1983; A.R. Gardner and Gardner 1975; Roy 1978). Bennum (1983) found that those who self-mutilated had more outwardly directed hostility than did nonmutilating patients with depression, but these groups did not differ in inwardly directed hostility. Simeon et al. (1992) reported that, compared with nonmutilating control subjects matched for personality disorder diagnoses, self-mutilating subjects had lifetime histories of greater aggression and sociopathy, and that the degree of self-mutilation correlated significantly with chronic anger. Indeed, Kernberg (1987) describes self-injury as an often revengeful enactment of an attempt to control the other.

Self-injuring inmates make up a unique subpopulation in which some of these associations are prominent. Although not extensively studied, it is well known that self-mutilation is a fairly common phenomenon in male prisoners, with an estimated rate around 5% according to one study (Toch 1975). The literature suggests that, in this population, self-injury is strongly associated with antisocial or other severe personality disorders (Hillbrand et al. 1994; Rada and James 1982; Virkkunen 1976). The self-injuring acts are typically moderately severe, such as serious slashing or head banging; swallowing of objects such as razor blades, light bulbs, or bedsprings; or insertion of foreign bodies into the urethra (Fulwiler et al. 1997; Haines and Williams 1997; Rada and James 1982), and medical attention is often necessary. Although the severity of these acts can border on the types of behaviors seen with major SIB, psychosis is rarely associated with self-mutilation in this population (13% in one randomly selected series [Fulwiler et al. 1997]), and schizophrenia is less likely in this population than was found in inmate control subjects in another series (Hillbrand et al. 1994).

Contagion of self-mutilating behavior in prisons has been reported, often for motives related to secondary gain (Rada and James 1982). In addition to the common motive of conscious manipulation (31% of total in one series [Fulwiler et al. 1997]), other common motives are similar to those previously described for other individuals engaging in impulsive SIB, such as the relief of mounting anxiety or tension (Fulwiler et al. 1997). Indeed, in a controlled study, self-mutilating prisoners demonstrated more anxiety, dysphoria, withdrawal, and rejection sensitivity (Fulwiler et al. 1997; Virkkunen 1976). It has been proposed that low environmental stimulation in the prison setting may precipitate self-injury in sensation-seeking sociopathic individuals (Virkkunen 1976). Onset of the self-injury may coincide with incarceration (Virkkunen 1976) or extensively predate it (Paulino and Krolikowski 1995; Rada and James 1982). Other correlates of self-injury in the prison population include mental retardation (Hillbrand et al. 1994; Rada and James 1982), outward-directed aggression and violence (Hillbrand et al. 1994; Virkkunen 1976), a history of childhood hyperactivity (Fulwiler et al. 1997), and deficient coping skills (Haines and Williams 1997). In summary, the combination of very severe underlying psychopathology, a frequent element of manipulation, and limited therapeutic resources in these settings all add to the challenge of understanding and treating self-injury in this unique group.

### Relationship to Trauma

Traumatic experiences commonly predate and appear to contribute to the development of impulsive self-injury. These experiences more typically occur in childhood, although adult trauma such as combat or rape has also been described as related to the onset of self-injury (Greenspan and Samuel 1989; Pitman 1990). Although numerous studies uncontestedly attest to the relationship between childhood trauma and SIB, the relevance and contribution of different types of childhood trauma (e.g., physical abuse, sexual abuse, neglect, or loss) is less clear and consistent. We review here some of the major descriptive studies in this area. More about the biology of trauma as it relates to self-injury can be found in Chapter 6, and the psychologic elaborations of trauma are discussed in Chapter 8.

In one large study of "habitual female self-mutilators," childhood abuse was noted in 62% of the subjects. Of these, 29% reported both sexual and physical abuse, 17% reported only sexual abuse, and 16% reported only physical abuse. The onset of the abuse was typically early, reported as early latency, and it often involved family members (Favazza and Conterio 1989). Indeed, abused and neglected children can begin to exhibit SIBs at a disturbingly early age. In a study of children aged 2.5–5 years who were abused or neglected, both self-mutilation and suicidal behavior were described (P.A. Rosenthal and Rosenthal 1984). In another study of somewhat older physically or sexually abused children, 41% exhibited self-mutilation such as head banging or self-biting (Green 1978).

One comprehensive study attempting to tease out the contribution of various factors to the genesis and perpetuation of self-destructive behaviors followed-up 74 individuals with personality disorder over a 4-year period (van der Kolk et al. 1991). A portion of this group had a history of self-mutilation, and within the self-mutilating group the incidence of major disruptions in parental care was 89% and the incidence of childhood trauma such as physical abuse, sexual abuse, or witnessing domestic violence was 79%. Sexual abuse most strongly predicted self-injury, which was also associated with younger age at the time of the abuse as well as with childhood chaos, separations, and neglect. Dissociative experiences also correlated with self-mutilation. Interestingly, neglect and separation from caregivers predicted continuation of the self-injury in the face of treatment efforts, leading the authors to postulate that the latter traumas impaired the capacity to form trusting, stable bonds with others that could then facilitate treatment change. Another study of inpatients with borderline personality disorder compared with control subjects with personality disorder similarly found that both parental sexual abuse and emotional neglect were significantly related to self-mutilation (Dubo et al. 1997).

The experience of heightening dissociation leading to self-injury is commonly described by these patients and is supported by several studies such as the one described above. However, some studies have failed to confirm the link between trauma, dissociation, and self-injury. Two recent studies using the same design, one of male and another of female borderline patients, compared self-mutilators with nonmutilators and found that all variables examined (physical abuse, sexual abuse, separations/losses, bonding, and dissociation) failed to discriminate the two groups (Zweig-Frank et al. 1994a, 1994b). The authors interpreted their results to mean that abuse and dissociation may not account for self-mutilation in personality disorder. However, other studies have found a powerful link between dissociation and self-injury. In a large study of female inpatients, self-mutilators displayed greater dissociation, alexithymia, and frequency of childhood sexual abuse than did nonmutilators (Zlotnick et al. 1996). Furthermore, alexithymia and dissociation were independently associated with self-mutilation, a very interesting finding suggesting that the inability to know and describe affective states is, in and of itself, a risk factor for translating these states into action and self-injuring. A second study of female inpatients with borderline personality disorder found self-mutilation to be the most powerful predictor of dissociation and that subjects who dissociated were more likely to report childhood abuse (Brodsky et al. 1995).

It seems clear that even though the exact correlates of impulsive self-injury in terms of types of childhood trauma may vary from patient to patient and study to study, the etiologic role of childhood trauma in a significant number of patients who engage in self-injury later in life is undeniable. The mediating factors are, probably, various trauma-induced or trauma-facilitated dysregulations with concomitant biologic underpinnings such as affective dysregulation, poor impulse control, dissociation, and poor modulation of aggression. By the same token, childhood trauma should not automatically be assumed in any patient with this type of self-injury, and clinicians are always cautioned against overeagerly searching for such a history.

Another type of childhood trauma that is at times associated with self-injury is early invasive physical trauma, such as mutilations or surgeries. In one study, R.J. Rosenthal et al. (1972) found that most self-injuring patients in their series had suffered serious illnesses, accidents, or surgeries before age 12, whereas none of the matched control subjects had had similar experiences.

## Assessment of Self-Injurious Behaviors

A thorough assessment of SIBs is, of course, the first step in understanding and therefore becoming able to intervene and treat these behaviors successfully. Our recommendation is that a simple inquiry about self-injury be incorporated into any initial psychiatric evaluation as routinely as any other list of psychiatric symptoms inquired about with patients. The single question "have you ever physically hurt yourself in any way?" can routinely follow inquiry about suicidal ideation, gestures, or attempts. A few specific examples of SIBs may be offered to supplement this question. This approach can help patients to come forward with information that they might feel too embarassed or otherwise reluctant to spontaneously reveal.

If patients acknowledge any SIB, a detailed history should then be obtained. A sensitive clinician must always be aware of the unspoken aspects of their communications, and patients might experience being asked about and giving their self-injury history as shameful, exhibitionistic, intrusive, or as a sign of interest on the part of the clinician. These experiences can always be explored with the patient; however, such concerns typically do not justify not learning the patient's self-injury story, and failure to elicit these details may be interpreted by the patient as indicating that the clinician does not know or care enough about these behaviors.

We present an overview of a standard history of SIBs that is also summarized in Table 1–2. The clinician should inquire about age of onset and course to the present, such as whether the behavior has been intermittent or continuous and what has been the longest period of time elapsed during which the patient did not engage in it. The frequency of the behavior, whether in number of episodes or total time spent daily, needs to be determined on a lifetime and a current basis. Any major or minor medical complications and interventions, such as infections, scars, stitches, fractures, or corrective surgery, should also be questioned. The chronicity, frequency, and medical sequalae taken together render an impression about the overall severity of each patient's self-injury.

---

**Table 1–2.** Evaluation of self-injurious behaviors

---

Inquiry about any history of self-injurious behaviors

Presence of suicidal ideation (any intent to die as a result of the behavior should be absent)

Temporal relationship to suicidality/suicidal behaviors

Lifetime and current frequency of self-injurious behavior (number of episodes or daily time spent)

Age of onset, course, longest period free of behavior, change over time

Medical complications or interventions

Motivations/emotional states/triggers leading up to the behavior

Aftermath of the behavior: immediate and subsequent

Preexisting urge/impulsivity

Dystonicity (wish to stop oneself)

Resistance (effort to stop oneself)

Control (success in stopping oneself)

Analgesia

Use of substances before and during the act

Family history of self-injurious behavior

Personal treatment history of self-injurious behavior (pharmacologic and psychotherapeutic)

---

The patient's subjective experience of the behavior is of equal importance. General questions about how patients understand and what they make of the behavior (their personal theories about it) are supplemented by more specific questions about the motivations, emotional states, interpersonal communications, and situational triggers related to the behavior. In addition, patients should be questioned about their wish to engage in the behavior (dystonicity), their efforts to resist it (resistance), and their ability to control it (control). One should also inquire whether the behavior is preceeded by any sense of an urge and how impulsive the act is (i.e., how much time usually elapses from when the self-injurious thought first occurs to when the act is executed). It is important to find out if patients are or become intoxicated with alcohol or drugs when they engage in self-injury. The experience of physical pain during the act and its meanings to the patient as well as the cues to stop are also important. A family history of SIBs is sometimes present and might suggest biologic predispositions or significant meanings of the behavior for the particular patient. The presence of suicidal ideation during the behavior must be inquired about, even if the act itself had no suicidal intent, and any temporal pattern between escalating SIB and suicidality should be clarified. Finally, past treatment history for these behaviors, whether directly or in the context of a more general therapy, must be thoroughly assessed to uncover any interventions, pharmacologic or psychotherapeutic, that have been helpful or detrimental. The degree to which patients were forthcoming or secretive about self-injury with previous clinicians is also of interest and may predict their future communication pattern. A complete evaluation of SIBs will enable the clinician to consider various appropriate treatment options, which are described in detail later in this book.

## References

American Psychiatric Association: Diagnostic and Statistical Manual of Mental Disorders, 4th Edition. Washington, DC, American Psychiatric Association, 1994

Arnold LM, McElroy SL, Mutasim DF, et al: Characteristics of 34 adults with psychogenic excoriation. J Clin Psychiatry 59:509–514, 1998

Azrin NH, Nunn RG: Habit reversal: a method of eliminating nervous habits and tics. Behav Res Ther 11:619–628, 1973

Bach-Y-Rita G: Habitual violence and self-mutilation. Am J Psychiatry 131:1018–1020, 1974

Bakwin H: Nail-biting in twins. Dev Med Child Neurol 13:304–307, 1971

Ballinger B: The prevalence of nail biting in normal and abnormal populations. Br J Psychiatry 117:445–446, 1970

Bennum I: Depression and hostility in self-mutilation. Suicide Life Threat Behav 13:71–84, 1983

Birch LB: The incidence of nail-biting among school-children. Br J Educ Psychol 25:123–128, 1955

Bodfish JM, Crawford TM, Powell SB, et al: Compulsions in adults with mental retardation: prevalence, phenomenology and comorbidity with stereotypy and self-injury. Am J Ment Retard 100:183–192, 1995

Brodsky BS, Cloitre M, Dulit RA: Relationship of dissociation to self-mutilation and childhood abuse in borderline personality disorder. Am J Psychiatry 152:1788–1792, 1995

Bryson Y, Sakati N, Nyhan WL, et al: Self-injurious behavior in the Cornelia de Lange syndrome. Am J Ment Defic 76:319–324, 1971

Christenson GA, Mackenzie TB, Mitchell JE: Characteristics of 60 adult chronic hair-pullers. Am J Psychiatry 148:365–370, 1991a

Christenson, GA, Pyle RL, Mitchell JE: Estimated lifetime prevalence of trichotillomania in college students. J Clin Psychiatry 52:415–417, 1991b

Christenson GA, Chernoff-Clementz E, Clementz BA: Personality and clinical characteristics in patients with trichotillomania. J Clin Psychiatry 53:407–413, 1992

Christenson GA, Ristvedt SL, MacKenzie TB: Identification of trichotillomania cue profiles. Behav Res Ther 31:315–320, 1993

Clark RA: Self-mutilation accompanying religious delusions. J Clin Psychiatry 42:243–245, 1981

Clarke DJ, Waters J, Corbett JA: Adults with Prader-Willi syndrome: abnormalities of sleep and behavior. J R Soc Med 82:21–24, 1989

Cohen LJ, Stein DJ, Simeon D, et al: Clinical profile, comorbidity and treatment history in 123 hair-pullers: a survey study. J Clin Psychiatry 36:319–326, 1995

Coons PM, Milstein V: Self-mutilation associated with dissociative disorders. Dissociation 3:81–87, 1990

DeMuth GW, Strain J, Lombardo-Mahar A: Self-amputation and restitution. Gen Hosp Psychiatry 5:25–30, 1983

Doran AR, Roy A, Wolkowitz OM: Self-destructive dermatoses. Psychiatr Clin North Am 8:291–298, 1985

Dubo ED, Zanarini MC, Lewis RE, et al: Childhood antecedents of self-destructiveness in borderline personality disorder. Can J Psychiatry 42:63–69, 1997

Dubovsky SL: "Experimental" self-mutilation. Am J Psychiatry 135:1240–1241, 1978

Favaro A, Santonastaso P: Impulsive and compulsive self-injurious behavior in bulimia nervosa: prevalence and psychological correlates. J Nerv Ment Dis 186:157–165, 1998

Favazza A: Why patients mutilate themselves. Hospital and Community Psychiatry 40:137–145, 1989

Favazza A: Bodies Under Siege: Self-Mutilation and Body Modification in Culture and Psychiatry, 2nd Edition. Baltimore, MD, The Johns Hopkins University Press, 1996

Favazza A: The coming of age of self-mutilation. J Nerv Ment Dis 186:259–268, 1998

Favazza A, Conterio K: Female habitual self-mutilators. Acta Psychiatr Scand 79:283–289, 1989

Favazza A, Rosenthal R: Varieties of pathological self-mutilation. Behav Neurol 3:77–85, 1990

Favazza A, Simeon D: Self-mutilation, in Impulsivity and Aggression. Edited by Hollander E and Stein DJ. Chichester, England, John Wiley and Sons, 1995

Favazza A, DeRosear L, Conterio K: Self-mutilation and eating disorders. Suicide Life Threat Behav 19:352–361, 1989

Fulwiler C, Forbes C, Santangelo SL, et al: Self-mutilation and suicide attempt: distinguishing features in prisoners. J Am Acad Psychiatry Law 25:69–77, 1997

Gardner AR, Gardner AJ: Self-mutilation, obsessionality, and narcissism. Br J Psychiatry 127:127–132, 1975

Gardner DL, Cowdry RW: Suicidal and parasuicidal behavior in borderline personality disorder. Psychiatr Clin North Am 8:389–403, 1985

Garfinkel PE, Moldofsky H, Garner DM: The heterogeneity of anorexia nervosa. Arch Gen Psychiatry 37:1036–1040, 1980

Goodhart S, Savitsky N: Self-mutilation in chronic encephalitis. Am J Med Sci 185:674–684, 1933

Graff H, Mallin R: The syndrome of the wrist cutter. Am J Psychiatry 124:36–42, 1967

Griffin JC, Williams DE, Stark MT, et al: Self-injurious behavior: a statewide prevalence survey of the extent and circumstances. Appl Res Ment Retard 7:105–116, 1986

Green AH: Self-destructive behavior in battered children. Am J Psychiatry 135:579–582, 1978

Greenspan GC, Samuel SE: Self-cutting after rape. Am J Psychiatry 146:789–790, 1989

Greilsheimer H, Groves JE: Male genital self-mutilation. Arch Gen Psychiatry 36:441–446, 1979

Gupta MA, Gupta AK, Haberman HF: Neurotic excoriations: a review and some new perspectives. Compr Psychiatry 27:381–386, 1986

Hadley NH: Fingernail Biting: Theory, Research, and Treatment. New York, Spectrum, 1984

Haines J, Williams CL: Coping and problem solving of self-mutilators. J Clin Psychology 53:177–186, 1997

Hillbrand M, Krystal JH, Sharpe KS, et al: Clinical predictors of self-mutilation in hospitalized forensic patients. J Nerv Ment Dis 182:9–13, 1994

Jankovic J: Orofacial and other self-mutilations, in Advances in Neurology: Facial Dyskinesias, Vol 49. Edited by Jankovic J. New York, Rowen Press, 1988, pp 365–381

Kafka JS: The body as transitional object: a psychoanalytic study of a self-mutilating patient. Br J Med Psychol 42:207–212, 1969

Kennedy BL, Feldman TB: Self-inflicted eye injuries: case presentations and a literature review. Hospital and Community Psychiatry 45:470–474, 1994

Kernberg O: The borderline self-mutilator. J Personal Disord 1:344–346, 1987

King BH: Self-injury by people with mental retardation: a compulsive behavior hypothesis. Am J Ment Retard 98:93–112, 1993

Krieger MJ, McAninch JW, Weimer SR: Self-performed bilateral orchiectomy in transsexuals. J Clin Psychiatry 43:292–293, 1982

Krishnan KRR, Davidson JRT, Guajardo C: Trichotillomania: a review. Compr Psychiatry 26:123–128, 1985

Leibenluft E, Gardner DL, Cowdry RW: The inner experience of the borderline self-mutilator. J Personal Disord 1:317–324, 1987

Leonard HL, Lenane MC, Swedo SE, et al: A double-blind comparison of clomipramine and desipramine treatment of severe onychophagia (nail biting). Arch Gen Psychiatry 48:821–827, 1991

Lesch M, Nyhan WL: A familial disorder of uric acid metabolism and central nervous system function. Am J Med 36:561–570, 1964

Massler M, Malone AJ: Nail-biting: a review. J Paediatr 36:523–531, 1950

Martin T, Gattaz WF: Psychiatric aspects of male genital self-mutilation. Psychopathology 24:170–178, 1991

McKerracher DW, Loughnane T, Watson RA: Self-mutilation in female psychopaths. Br J Psychiatry 114:829–832, 1968

Menninger K: A psychoanalytic study of the significance of self-mutilation. Psychoanal Q 4:408–466, 1935

Menninger K: Man Against Himself. New York, Harcourt Brace World, 1938

Mitchell JE, Boutacoff LI, Hatsukami D, et al: Laxative abuse as a variant of bulimia. J Nerv Ment Dis 174:174–176, 1986

Moskovitz RA, Byrd T: Rescuing the angel within: PCP-related self-enucleation. Psychosomatics 4:402–406, 1983

Nakaya M: On background factors of male genital self-mutilation. Psychopathology 29:242–248, 1996

Oranje AP, Peereboom-Wynia JDR, De Raeymaecker DMJ: Trichotillomania in childhood. J Am Acad Dermatol 15:614–619, 1986

Pao PN: The syndrome of delicate self-cutting. Br J Med Psychology 42:195–206, 1969

Parkin JR, Eagles JM: Bloodletting in bulimia nervosa. Br J Psychiatry 162:246-248, 1993

Pattison EM, Kahan J: The deliberate self-harm syndrome. Am J Psychiatry 140:867–872, 1983

Paulino AFG, Krolikowski FJ: Insertion of foreign bodies into the abdominal cavity. Am J Forensic Med Pathol 16:48–50, 1995

Pennington LA: The incidence of nail-biting among adults. Am J Psychiatry 102:241–244, 1945

Pitman RK: Self-mutilation in combat related post-traumatic stress disorder. Am J Psychiatry 147:123–124, 1990

Pitman RK, Green RC, Jenike MA, et al: Clinical comparison of Tourette's disorder and obsessive-compulsive disorder. Am J Psychiatry 144:1166–1171, 1987

Prader A, Labhart A, Willi H: Ein syndrom von adipositas, kleinwuchs, kryptochismus und oligophrenie nach myatonieartigem zustand im neugeborenenalter. Schweizerische Medizinische Wochenschrift 86:1260–1261, 1956

Rada RT, James W: Urethral insertion of foreign bodies: a report of contagious self-mutilation in a maximum-security hospital. Arch Gen Psychiatry 39:423–429, 1982

Reti-Gyorgy A, Palyi M, Nagy A: Giant "cast" benzoar in the stomach removable only by surgery. Orv Hetil 138:149–151, 1997

Robertson MM: The Gilles de la Tourette syndrome: the current status. Br J Psychiatry 154:147–169, 1989

Robertson MM, Trimble MR, Lees A: Self-injurious behavior and the Gilles de la Tourette syndrome: a clinical study and review of the literature. Psychol Med 19:611–625, 1989

Rosenthal PA, Rosenthal S: Suicidal behavior by preschool children. Am J Psychiatry 141:520–525, 1984

Rosenthal RJ, Rinzler C, Walsh R, et al: Wrist-cutting syndrome. Am J Psychiatry 128:1363–1368, 1972

Rothbaum BO, Shaw L, Morris R, et al: The prevalence of trichotillomania in a college freshman population. J Clin Psychiatry 54:72, 1993

Rothenberger A: Psychopharmacological treatment of self-injurious behavior in autism. Acta Paediopsychiatr 56:99–104, 1993

Roy A: Self-mutilation. Br J Med Psychol 51:201–203, 1978

Schaffer CB, Carrll J, Abramowitz SI: Self-mutilation and the borderline personality. J Nerv Ment Dis 170:468–473, 1982

Schepis C, Failla P, Siraguse M, et al: Skin-picking: the best cutaneous feature in the recognition of Prader-Willi syndrome. Int J Dermatol 33:866–867, 1994

Shear CS, Nyhan WL, Kirman BH et al: Self-mutilative behaviour as a feature of the de Lange syndrome. J Pediatr 78:506–509, 1971

Simeon D, Stanley B, Frances A, et al: Self-mutilation in personality disorders: psychological and biological correlates. Am J Psychiatry 149:221–226, 1992

Simeon D, Stein DJ, Hollander E: Depersonalization disorder and self-injurious behavior. J Clin Psychiatry 56(suppl):36–39, 1995

Simeon D, Cohen LJ, Stein DJ, et al: Comorbid self-injurious behaviors in 71 female hair-pullers: a survey study. J Nerv Ment Dis 185:117–119, 1997a

Simeon D, Stein DJ, Gross S, et al: A double-blind trial of fluoxetine in pathologic skin-picking. J Clin Psychiatry 58:341–347, 1997b

Simeon D, Gross S, Guralnik O, et al: Feeling unreal: 30 cases of DSM-III-R depersonalization disorder. Am J Psychiatry 154:1107–1113, 1997c

Simpson MA: Self-mutilation and suicide, in Suicidology: Contemporary Developments. Edited by Schneidman ES. New York, Grune & Stratton, 1976

Singh NN, Pulman RM: Self-injury in the de Lange syndrome. J Ment Defic Res 23:79–81, 1979

Soriano JL, O'Sullivan RL, Baer L, et al: Trichotillomaina and self-esteem: a survey of 62 female hair-pullers. J Clin Psychiatry 57:77–82, 1996

Stanley MA, Swann, C, Bowers, TC, et al: A comparison of clinical features in trichotillomania and obsessive-compulsive disorder. Behav Res Ther 30:39–44, 1992

Stein DJ, Keating J, Zar HJ, et al: A survey of the phenomenology and pharmacotherapy of compulsive and impulsive-aggressive symptoms in Prader-Willi syndrome. J Neuropsych Clin Neurosci 6:23–29, 1994

Stein DJ, Simeon D, Cohen LJ, et al: Trichotillomania and obsessive-compulsive disorder. J Clin Psychiatry 56(suppl):28–34, 1995

Stone MH: The Fate of Borderline Patients: Successful Outcome and Psychiatric Practice. New York, Guilford, 1990, pp 61–63

Stroud JD: Hair loss in children. Pediatr Clin North Am 30:641–657, 1983

Swedo SE: Trichotillomania, in The Obsessive-Compulsive Related Disorders. Edited by Hollander E. Washington, DC, American Psychiatric Press, 1993

Swedo SE, Rapoport JL: Annotation: trichotillomania. J Child Psychol Psychiatry 32:401–409, 1991

Swedo SE, Leonard HL, Rapoport JL et al: A double-blind comparison of clomipramine and desipramine in the treatment of trichotillomania (hair-pulling). N Engl J Med 321:497–501, 1989a

Swedo SE, Rapoport JL, Leonard H, et al: Obsessive-compulsive disorder in children and adolescents. Arch Gen Psychiatry 46:335–341, 1989b

Thompson JN, Abraham TK: Male genital mutilation after paternal death. Br Med J 287:727–728, 1983

Toch H: Men in Crisis: Human Breakdowns in Prison. Chicago, IL, Aldine Press, 1975

van der Kolk BA, Perry JC, Herman JL: Childhood origins of self-destructive behavior. Am J Psychiatry 148:1665–1671, 1991

Virkkunen M: Self-mutilation in antisocial personality disorder. Acta Psychiatr Scand 54:347–352, 1976

Wechsler D: Incidence and significance of fingernail biting in children. Psychoanal Rev 18:201–209, 1931

Winchel RM: Trichotillomania: presentation and treatment. Psychiatr Ann 22:84–88, 1992

Winchel RM, Stanley M: Self-injurious behavior: a review of the behavior and biology of self-mutilation. Am J Psychiatry 148:306–317, 1991

Winchel RM, Jones JS, Molcho A, et al: Rating the severity of trichotillomania: methods and problems. Psychopharmacol Bull 28:457–462, 1992

Zlotnick C, Shea MT, Pearlstein T, et al: The relationship between dissociative symptoms, alexithymia, impulsivity, sexual abuse and self-mutilation. Compr Psychiatry 37:12–16, 1996

Zweig-Frank H, Paris J, Grizder J: Psychological risk factors and self-mutilation in male patients with borderline personality disorder. Can J Psychiatry 39:266–268, 1994a

Zweig-Frank H, Paris J, Grizder J: Psychological risk factors for dissociation and self-mutilation in female patients with borderline personality disorder. Can J Psychiatry 39:529–264, 1994b

# CHAPTER 2

# Stereotypic Self-Injurious Behaviors
## Neurobiology and Psychopharmacology

Dan J. Stein, M.B.
Dana J.H. Niehaus, M.B.

## Introduction

Self-injurious behaviors (SIBs) are seen in several disorders that are usually first diagnosed in infancy or childhood. Stereotypic movement disorder (SMD) with SIB is commonly seen in patients with mental retardation. In addition, SIBs are often encountered in several specific syndromes typically characterized by mental retardation, including Lesch-Nyhan, Cornelia de Lange, and Prader-Willi syndromes. Finally, SIBs are seen in pervasive developmental disorders such as autism. In this chapter we focus on the neurochemical systems that may underlie these various forms of SIB and at the same time discuss their psychopharmacologic management.

## Stereotypic Movement Disorder

SIBs in patients with mental retardation and other developmental disorders may fall within the diagnostic category of SMD, which is characterized by repetitive, seemingly driven, but nonfunctional motor behavior. Examples include body rocking, hand waving, head banging, and skin picking. The DSM-IV (American Psychiatric Association 1994) provides a subtype of "with self-injurious behavior" to be used when bodily damage requires medical treatment.

Several DSM-IV criteria for SMD address the severity of the behavior—"markedly interferes with normal activities or results in self-inflicted bodily injury that requires medical treatment" (American Psychiatric Association 1994, p. 121). In patients with mental retardation, the behavior must be sufficiently severe to be a focus of treatment and must persist for at least 4 weeks. The DSM-IV also states that these behaviors should not be better accounted for by the compulsions of obsessive-compulsive disorder (OCD), the stereotypies of pervasive developmental disorder, or the tics of Tourette's syndrome.

SIBs in patients with mental retardation and other developmental disorders may not always meet these rather strict DSM-IV criteria for SMD. Nevertheless, evidence has shown that stereotyped, self-injurious, and compulsive behaviors appear to be correlated in such patients (Bodfish et al. 1995). The relatively large body of work on the pathogenesis and treatment of stereotypic behaviors in this population may be useful in understanding and managing such behavior. A range of theories has been put forward to explain stereotypic behavior in patients with mental retardation, including extension of behaviors that are normal at an early developmental level (Berkson 1983), arousal modulation in response to over- and understimulating environments (Leuba 1955), reinforcement by environmental events, and neurobiologic dysfunction (Cooper and Dourish 1990). These different theories have been integrated in different ways (Guess and Carr 1991; King 1993; Lovaas et al. 1987; Oliver 1983), and they have been crucial in assessing and treating stereotypic behaviors.

Neurobiologic theories of SMD have drawn on preclinical work, on studies of patients with neurologic lesions, and on research on psychiatric disorders that are characterized by repetitive nonfunctional symptoms. Thus, evidence for the involvement of frontal-basal ganglia circuitry in stereotypic behavior emerges from preclinical studies of frontal and striatal lesions (Ridley 1994) as well as from research in patients with OCD and Tourette's syndrome. This work has also investigated the role of different neurotransmitter systems in stereotypic movements and overlaps with the psychopharmacologic focus of this chapter.

## Mental Retardation

Reports of the incidence of SIBs in patients with mental retardation range from 3% to 46% (Bodfish et al. 1995; Winchel and Stanley 1991). Head banging, head and body hitting, eye gouging, biting, and scratching are the most common of these behaviors (King 1993). Such behaviors may cause permanent and disabling tissue damage and may sometimes be life threatening. For example, severe head banging or hitting may lead to cuts, bleeding, infection, retinal detachment, and blindness. The incidence of SIBs in patients with mental retardation is dependent on several factors that vary within this heterogeneous population, including extent of cognitive impairment (King 1993) and institutionalization status (Winchel and Stanley 1991).

Given the heterogeneity of patients with mental retardation it is possible that SIBs in different patients reflect entirely different neurobiologic mechanisms. Nevertheless, it may be argued that specific behaviors shared across diagnostic categories are mediated by similar neurobiologic mechanisms (Van Praag et al. 1986). Several neurochemical systems have been hypothesized to play a role in the mediation of SIB in a range of different patients with mental retardation. In this section we focus on the possible roles of the neurotransmitters serotonin and dopamine and also on the opioid system.

### Serotonin

Both preclinical research and clinical studies have supported a significant correlation between abnormal serotonin function and increased impulsive aggression, including self-directed impulsive-aggressive behaviors (Stein et al. 1993; Van Praag et al. 1986). Furthermore, increasing evidence shows that the serotonin system plays a significant role in OCD and other disorders characterized by repetitive behaviors, with serotonin reuptake inhibitors showing efficacy preferentially in the pharmacotherapy of OCD (Stein 1996; Zohar and Insel 1987). Thus, it is tempting to hypothesize a role for serotonin in the mediation of SIB in mental retardation. It has been argued that there is phenomenologic evidence of similarities between SIBs in patients with mental retardation and symptoms in patients with OCD (King 1993). Furthermore, in patients with mental retardation, significant positive associations exist among the occurence of self-injury, stereotypy, and compulsions (Bodfish et al. 1995). Nevertheless, relatively few studies have directly explored the role of serotonin in the mediation of SIBs in mental retardation.

Evidence for the value of serotonin reuptake inhibitors in the treatment of SIBs in mental retardation is increasing, however. A retrospective review of antidepressants in patients with mental retardation suggested that response of SIBs was higher for serotonin reuptake inhibitors and was not predicted by comorbid depressive symptoms (Mikkelson et al. 1997). Indeed, both open (Cook et al. 1992; Garber et al. 1992; Hellings et al. 1996;

Markowitz 1992; Ricketts et al. 1993) and controlled (Lewis et al. 1996) studies have confirmed the efficacy of serotonin reuptake inhibitors in the treatment of SIBs in patients with mental retardation.

Although this research is certainly consistent with a role for serotonin in the mediation of SIBs in mental retardation, questions remain about whether the effects of these agents are not "downstream" to their primary actions and about their specificity. Several methodologies are now available for delineating different aspects of serotonin dysfunction in psychiatric patients (Coccaro et al. 1989), and the "pharmacological dissection" strategy of comparing response to clomipramine with that to desipramine has been useful in showing that serotonin plays a specific role in several disorders characterized by unwanted repetitive behaviors (Leonard et al. 1991; Swedo et al. 1989). We look forward to similar work being undertaken in patients with mental retardation and SIB.

It may be noted here that other agents with serotonergic effects have also been studied for the treatment of SIB in patients with mental retardation. 5-Hydroxytryptamine (5-HT) has been shown useful in only a minority of open studies (Winchel and Stanley 1991). Buspirone (15–45 mg/ day), a $5-HT_{1A}$ agonist, was somewhat effective in small groups of adults with mental retardation and SIB (Ratey et al. 1989; Ricketts et al. 1994). Eltoprazine, a selective $5-HT_{1A}$ and $5-HT_{1B}$ agonist (Kohen 1993; Tiihonen et al. 1993; Verhoeven et al. 1992), has provided conflicting evidence for efficacy.

Several agents such as lithium and β-blockers have multiple neurotransmitter effects, including serotonergic effects. Although early studies in this area suffered from methodologic flaws, lithium has long been used with some apparent success in the treatment of SIB and aggressive behaviors in patients with mental retardation (Lapierre and Reesal 1986; Osman and Loschen 1992; Wickham and Reed 1987). More recently, propranolol (90–410 mg/day) was reported to reduce SIB and aggression in five of six patients with mental retardation (Luchins and Dojka 1989). Furthermore, in a controlled study, pindolol (40 mg/day) was significantly more effective than placebo in 14 patients with mental retardation (Ratey and Lindem 1991).

## Dopamine

As with serotonin, both preclinical and clinical studies support a role for dopamine in the mediation of stereotypic and compulsive symptoms. Of particular relevance to developmental disorders is the hypothesis that early destruction of dopaminergic neurons in preclinical models may lead to hypersensitivity of D1 receptors, with increased stereotypic behavior after administration of dopamine agonists later in life (Breese et al. 1984).

In addition, both preclinical and clinical studies demonstrate significant interactions between the serotonin and the dopamine systems (Kapur and Remington 1996). A particularly significant finding in the OCD literature, for example, has been that patients with comorbid tics are more frequently resistant to treatment with serotonin reuptake inhibitors but may respond to augmentation of these agents with dopamine blockers (McDougle et al. 1994).

Relatively little direct work has been done on the dopamine system in patients with mental retardation and SIB. Nevertheless, recent work on specific syndromes such as Lesch-Nyhan syndrome (see below) supports the importance of this system in mediating SIBs in some patients with mental retardation. Furthermore, dopamine blockers are often successfully used to manage SIBs in patients with mental retardation (Mikkelson 1986). Indeed, in an open trial, fluphenazine (2–8 mg/day) led to clinical improvement in these symptoms in 11 of 15 patients with mental retardation (Gualtieri and Schroeder 1989).

Preliminary evidence suggests that atypical neuroleptics, which have both dopaminergic and serotonergic effects, may also be useful in self-injurious and other target symptoms in patients with mental retardation (Cohen and Underwood 1994; Rubin 1997). Given their apparently favorable side effect profile, controlled trials with these agents are warranted.

## Opioids

Several authors have suggested that the opioid system plays a crucial role in mediating SIBs (Herman 1990; Sandman 1990). In preclinical work, opioid agonists may induce autoaggression, and opioid antagonists may be particularly effective in reducing self-injurious stereotypies in younger animals (Cronin et al. 1986). Indeed, it has been suggested that excessive opioid activity underlies SIBs (Herman et al. 1989). However, an alternative hypothesis emphasizes that pain associated with SIB results in release of brain endorphins and draws a parallel between such endogenous release of endorphins and addiction to an exogenous substance (Cataldo and Harris 1982).

Sandman (1988) found increased plasma enkephalin levels in patients with mental retardation compared with those found in normal control subjects. Although these findings may support the excessive opioid hypothesis, it is also possible that decreased endogenous brain opioids ultimately leads to compensatory overproduction (Pies and Popli 1995). It has also been argued, however, that opioid effects on self-injury may primarily be mediated via the dopamine or serotonin system (Winchel and Stanley 1991).

Some evidence has shown that the opiate antagonists naloxone and naltrexone lead to a reduction in frequency of self-injury in different patient populations, including those with mental retardation (Osman and Loschen 1992; Winchel and Stanley 1991). However, the total number of patients in such studies is relatively small and the study designs have been criticized (Pies and Popli 1995; Willemsen-Swinkels et al. 1995). Indeed, in a recent placebo-controlled study of 32 subjects with mental retardation, SIB, and/or autism, naltrexone (50 mg/day) failed to have an effect on SIB and increased the incidence of stereotypic behavior (Willemsen-Swinkels et al. 1995). Although this finding does not entirely rule out a role for the opioid system, it further emphasizes the need for caution in drawing conclusions from open trials of treatment for SIB in this population.

## Other Systems

SIBs may vary in women with mental retardation according to the stage of menstrual cycle. Taylor et al. (1993), for example, found that fluctuations in level of self-injury were associated with early and late follicular phases. Although data are insufficient at present for a specific association between SIB and hormonal factors, such an association deserves further study.

The use of benzodiazepines to treat SIBs in mental retardation has not been well studied. Further attention should perhaps be paid to the role of the γ-aminobutyric acid (GABA) system in SIB in mental retardation (Breese et al. 1967; Kopin 1981). From a clinical viewpoint, however, the possible risks of disinhibition and of dependence should be borne in mind when considering the use of these agents.

The anticonvulsant valproic acid was effective in reducing SIB and aggression in 12 of 18 patients with mental retardation and affective symptoms in a 2-year open trial (Kastner et al. 1993). Positive response to valproate was associated with a past history of seizure disorder. Again, the possible use of anticonvulsants for SIBs in a subgroup of patients with mental retardation seems a useful avenue for further research.

Indeed, although the focus of this section is primarily on biologic mechanisms and pharmacotherapies that cross diagnostic boundaries, given the heterogeneity of mental retardation further work on subgroups of patients with mental retardation and SIBs is necessary. In the next section, we consider some particularly interesting subgroups—several discrete syndromes characterized by SIB, such as Lesch-Nyhan, Cornelia de Lange, and Prader-Willi syndromes.

## Syndromes with Self-Injurious Behavior

### *Lesch-Nyhan Syndrome*

Lesch-Nyhan syndrome (LNS) is an X-linked recessive disorder of purine synthesis. Patients present with hyperuricemia and neuropsychiatric symptoms including spasticity, choreoathetosis, dystonia, mental retardation, aggression, and SIB (Lesch and Nyhan 1964). The SIBs are dramatic and consist primarily of finger and lip biting, although head banging, tongue biting, eye and/or nose poking, and self-scratching also occur (Nyhan 1976; Shear et al. 1971).

Both the biochemical abnormality (virtual absence of hypoxanthine phosphoribosyltransferase [HPRT]) and the underlying genetic defect (a mutation of the HPRT locus located at q26-28 of the X chromosome) are well identified. However, the mechanisms underlying neuropsychiatric symptoms are less clear. Nevertheless, the biochemical systems implicated include the dopaminergic and serotonergic systems. Early postmortem findings in three patients with LNS demonstrated dramatically reduced levels of dopamine, homovanillic acid, and dopa decarboxylase in the basal ganglia (Lloyd et al. 1981), placing particular emphasis on the dopamine system. Preclinical studies with HPRT-deficient models (Dunnett et al. 1989; Jinnah et al. 1994) and clinical studies of neurotransmitters and metabolite levels in patients with the disorder (Lake and Ziegler 1977; Silverstein et al. 1985) support the importance of dopaminergic mediation of symptoms. Most recently, volumetric magnetic resonance imaging (MRI) and positron-emission tomography (PET) techniques have documented reduced caudate volume and reduced dopamine transporters in caudate and putamen (Wong et al. 1996) as well as decreased dopa decarboxylase activity and dopamine storage throughout the dopaminergic system in LNS (Ernst et al. 1996).

It is interesting to note that although patients with both LNS and Parkinson's disease demonstrate decreased dopamine neurons and motoric symptoms, there are important differences between them. Parkinson's disease, for example, is characterized by diminished motor output, whereas LNS is characterized by uncontrolled and exaggerated motor activity. These differences are likely to reflect the importance of the developmental stage at which dopaminergic deficits occur (Breese et al. 1984).

Although dopamine supersensitivity has also been hypothesized to play a role in SIB in LNS (Goldstein et al. 1986), and dopamine blockers have been used for their treatment, long-term treatment with these agents is not of clear benefit in LNS (Anderson and Ernst 1994; Watts et al. 1982).

It is possible that, in LNS, reorganization of the cortical-basal ganglia-thalamic pathways occurs during development (Ernst et al. 1996). Further understanding of the developmental neurobiology underlying this syndrome is therefore needed.

Researchers have also focused on the serotonin and other systems in LNS. Patients with LNS have slightly increased putamen serotonin and 5-hydroxyindoleacetic acid (5-HIAA) levels (Lloyd et al. 1981) and increased cerebrospinal fluid 5-HIAA levels (Jankovic et al. 1988). Early reports suggested that 5-HT (1–8mg/kg) was useful in the treatment of SIBs in LNS (Mizuno and Yugari 1974, 1975). However, only a minority of subsequent studies have confirmed this finding (Winchel and Stanley 1991). GABA systems may also be postulated to play a role in LNS (Kopin 1981), but again this hypothesis has not translated into successful pharmacotherapeutic strategies.

## Cornelia de Lange Syndrome

Cornelia de Lange syndrome is a rare congenital disorder characterized by a distinctive appearance and mental retardation. Patients with Cornelia de Lange syndrome manifest excessive grooming behavior (hand licking and hair stroking) and SIBs including head slapping and self-scratching (Bryson et al. 1971; Johnson et al. 1976; Shear et al. 1971; Singh and Pulman 1979).

Favazza (1987) noted phenomenologic similarities between the excessive grooming in Cornelia de Lange syndrome and preclinical dopamine agonist–induced stereotypies. Nevertheless, little direct research supports a dopamine hypothesis of this syndrome. Indeed, its underlying neurobiology remains relatively poorly understood.

In an early study, patients with Cornelia de Lange syndrome were found to have reduced whole-blood serotonin levels (Greenberg and Coleman 1973). Several possible mechanisms underlying this finding were considered, including a dysfunction in serotonin metabolism, failure to bind to platelets, or transporter abnormalities. Again, however, putative serotonin dysfunction may simply reflect dysfunction in other systems.

## Prader-Willi Syndrome

Prader-Willi syndrome is a congenital disorder that affects approximately 1 in 10,000 newborns and is one of the five most common abnormalities seen in birth defect clinics (Holm 1981; Prader et al. 1956). Prader-Willi syndrome is associated with marked hyperphagia and is the most common dysmorphic form of obesity. It is characterized by behavioral disturbances, mental retardation, sleep disturbances, neonatal hypotonia, and hypogonadism.

Behavioral disturbances in Prader-Willi syndrome include compulsive self-mutilation, impulsive temper outbursts, and classical obsessive-compulsive behaviors (Clarke et al. 1989; Stein et al. 1994b). Behavioral symptoms have considerable impact on caretakers and require extensive resources for their management (Greenswag 1987). SIBs are common and not necessarily associated with cognitive impairment (Stein et al. 1994b); these include skin and nose picking, nail biting, lip biting, and hair pulling (Stein et al. 1994b). Patients frequently have chronic skin sores (Schepis et al. 1994).

Abnormalities of chromosome 15 have been implicated in the etiology of Prader-Willi syndrome, and recent research using cytogenetic and molecular techniques suggests that identification of a specific genetic basis is possible in most patients (Mascari et al. 1992). In about 70% of patients a cytogenetically visible deletion can be detected in the paternally derived chromosome 15 (15q11q13), whereas in about 20% of patients both copies of chromosome 15 are inherited from the mother (maternal uniparental disomy) (Mascari et al. 1992).

Genotype-phenotype correlations in 167 patients with this syndrome found no significant difference in skin picking between patients with and those without a chromosomal deletion (Gillessen-Kaesbach et al. 1995). Nevertheless, the abnormal gene product in Prader-Willi syndrome may ultimately provide crucial information on a possible etiology for the SIB that is characteristic of these patients.

The possibility of using serotonergic drugs to treat Prader-Willi syndrome is raised by the role of serotonin and the efficacy of serotonergic agents in appetite control and eating disorders (Curzon 1990; Jimerson et al. 1990), compulsive skin picking (Stein et al. 1992; Stout 1990), impulsive-aggression, and obsessive-compulsive–related disorders. A double-blind trial of fenfluramine showed that this agent was useful for weight loss and other-directed aggressive behavior in patients with Prader-Willi syndrome but did not affect SIB (Selikowitz et al. 1990). However, the selective serotonin reuptake inhibitor fluoxetine has been described as useful for SIBs in several cases of Prader-Willi syndrome (Hellings and Warnock 1994; Warnock and Kestenbaum 1992), and a survey of caretakers suggested that serotonin reuptake inhibitors may be helpful for both impulsive-aggressive and compulsive symptoms in some patients (Stein et al. 1994b).

There is little controlled work supporting the use of other psychotropic agents in Prader-Willi syndrome. Opioid antagonists have been reported to decrease appetite in some patients (Kyriakides et al. 1980), but controlled work has not supported their efficacy (Zlotkin et al. 1986). From a neuroanatomic perspective, several authors have provided evidence for possible hypothalamic-pituitary dysfunction (Fiser et al. 1974), but again further work is needed to extend these findings and to determine the relationship of this dysfunction with behavioral symptoms. Indeed, little is presently understood about the underlying neurobiology of self-injury and other behavioral symptoms in this fascinating disorder.

## Autism

Autistic disorder (or classical autism) is a pervasive developmental disorder characterized by impairment in social interactions, communication deficits, and restrictive and stereotyped behaviors. Stereotyped SIBs are common in patients with this disorder and may also be seen in other pervasive developmental disorders that do not meet the narrower criteria for autistic disorder (Rothenberger 1993). Common forms of SIB in autism include hand/wrist biting, head banging, self-scratching, self-hitting, self-pinching, and hair pulling.

It has been argued that repetitive behaviors in autism cannot simply be subsumed under the banner of OCD (Baron-Cohen 1989). Indeed, compared with patients with OCD, adults with autism had a different range of repetitive symptoms; they were more likely to demonstrate repetitive ordering, hoarding, touching, tapping, rubbing, and SIBs (McDougle et al. 1995). Nevertheless, it may be postulated that at least some similarities exist in the underlying neurobiologic mediation of autism and OCD. Certainly, there appear to be serotonergic abnormalities in autism. Many studies have found elevated platelet serotonin levels (Anderson et al. 1987; Cook 1990); neuroendocrine challenge studies with serotonergic agents have indicated reduced serotonergic responsivity (Hoshino et al. 1984; McBride et al. 1989); and a tryptophan-depletion study found that autism resulted in increased SIB, motor stereotypies, and anxiety (McDougle et al. 1996b).

Despite early reports of the efficacy of fenfluramine in open trials in autism, subsequent controlled trials were disappointing (Campbell et al. 1988; Leventhal et al. 1993; Stern et al. 1990). However, both open (Cook et al. 1992; Hellings et al. 1996; McDougle et al. 1992) and placebo-controlled (McDougle et al. 1996a) trials with serotonin reuptake inhibitors have demonstrated efficacy in reducing symptoms such as SIBs in autism. Furthermore, the serotonin reuptake inhibitor clomipramine was more effective than the noradrenergic reuptake inhibitor desipramine in autism (Gordon et al. 1993). Nevertheless, not all studies of these agents have been positive (Sanchez et al. 1996).

Other neurochemical systems may also play a role in the mediation of SIBs in autism. A PET study demonstrated reduced dopaminergic activity in the anterior medial prefrontal cortex (Ernst et al. 1996). Controlled trials have demonstrated that dopamine blockers (like serotonin reuptake inhibitors) are effective in about 50% of patients with autism for target symptoms including SIBs (Anderson et al. 1989; Perry et al. 1989). Clinical experience indicates that in cases in which a medication is ineffective for autism, an agent from a different class of medication may be useful (McBride et al. 1996). The atypical neuroleptics, with their combined dopaminergic and serotonergic effects, also deserve further study (Rothenberger 1993; Zuddas et al. 1996).

Panskepp (1979) suggested that increased brain opioid activity might be involved in mediating the various symptoms of autism. Other authors have also emphasized a role for the opioid system in autism (Campbell et al. 1993; Chamberlain and Herman 1990). However, studies of opioid levels in autism have been inconsistent (Willemsen-Swinkels et al. 1995). Furthermore, despite promising open trials, the effect of opioid blockers on target symptoms, including SIBs, in autism has been disappointing in controlled studies (Willemsen-Swinkels et al. 1995).

The neuroanatomy of autism has also received increasing attention in recent years. Preliminary postmortem studies have found abnormalities in the cerebellum and limbic system, including the hippocampus and amygdala (Bauman 1991; Rapin 1997). Neurophysiologic research has demonstrated various abnormalities including aberrant processing in the frontal association cortex (Dunn 1994; Minshew 1991). Early work with pneumoencephalography suggested left temporal horn dilatation and an early MRI study found hypoplasia of the posterior cerebellar vermis, but later studies have been inconsistent (Bailey et al. 1996). Functional brain imaging studies to date are also inconsistent, although perhaps suggestive of dysfunction in the association cortex (Horwitz and Rumsey 1994; Minshew 1991). Clearly, much work remains to be done to understand the neuroanatomy of SIB in autism and to integrate behavioral and biologic findings in this disorder (Bailey et al. 1996).

Although many medical disorders may lead to autism, a specific association is not typical (Rapin 1997). Increasingly, however, there is promise for delineating the specific, albeit multiple, genetic factors underlying the disorder (McBride et al. 1996). Interestingly, preliminary evidence indicates a familial link with Tourette's syndrome (Comings and Comings

1991). Most recently, a possible link to the serotonin transporter gene has been suggested (Cook et al. 1997). Such work may ultimately lead to a clearer understanding of the neurobiology of autism and self-injury and to specific therapeutic interventions.

## Conclusion

We have described SIBs in several disorders that usually present in childhood. Although these disorders are heterogenous, certain consistent themes appeared throughout the discussion (Table 2–1). In particular, evidence often indicates that the serotonin and dopamine neurotransmitter systems mediate SIBs, and serotonin reuptake inhibitors and dopamine blockers have been effective in their treatment. Although other systems, such as the opioid system, have also been postulated to play a role in the mediation of SIBs in developmental disorders, there is less evidence of this available. Future research will need to return to the issue of heterogeneity, exploring the differing role of these neurochemical systems in different developmental disorders and in the different subtypes of each of these disorders.

**Table 2–1.** Selected controlled pharmacotherapy studies of self-injurious behaviors in developmental disorders

| Study | Disorder | Pharmacotherapy | Result |
|-------|----------|-----------------|--------|
| Selikowitz et al. 1990 | Prader-Willi syndrome | Fenfluramine | Ineffective |
| Ratey and Lindem 1991 | Mental retardation | Pindolol | Effective |
| Lewis et al. 1996 | Mental retardation | Clomipramine | Effective |
| Willemsen-Swinkels et al. 1995 | Mental retardation with autism and/ or self-injurious behavior | Naltrexone | Ineffective |
| Campbell et al. 1993 | Autism | Naltrexone | Ineffective |
| Stern et al. 1990 | Autism | Fenfluramine | Ineffective |
| Campbell et al. 1988 | Autism | Fenfluramine | Ineffective |
| Leventhal et al. 1993 | Autism | Fenfluramine | Ineffective |
| McDougle et al. 1996a | Autism | Fluvoxamine | Effective |
| Gordon et al. 1993 | Autism | Clomipramine | Effective |
| Anderson et al. 1989 | Autism | Haloperidol | Effective |
| Perry et al. 1989 | Autism | Haloperidol | Effective |

Unfortunately, given the complexity of the neurobiology of behavior, our current understanding seems relatively superficial. The data rarely point to a specific pathogenic mechanism underlying SIB in developmental disorders—systems that are "downstream" from those under study may ultimately be important. In addition, interactions between different neurotransmitter systems make too specific a focus on any one system overly simplistic. Nevertheless, it is likely that the genetic and biochemical underpinnings of some of the disorders discussed in this chapter will eventually be understood much more clearly. Hopefully, such advances will contribute to a more specific understanding of the pathogenesis of SIB.

Several authors have pointed to the need for improving the methodology of pharmacotherapy studies of SIBs in mental retardation (Farber 1987; Gualtieri and Schroeder 1989; Winchel and Stanley 1991). We have noted several occasions on which promising open data have not been confirmed by carefully controlled studies. Fortunately, the safety and efficacy of serotonin reuptake inhibitors have been well researched in a number of disorders, and therefore these are particularly useful treatment options at present. In clinical practice, such agents need to be combined with appropriate behavioral and milieu interventions. The atypical neuroleptics may have a particularly promising role in the treatment of SIBs in developmental disorders and deserve careful controlled study in the future. Long-term pharmacotherapy studies are also needed.

In this chapter, space has precluded a thorough exploration of the phenomenology and psychology of SIBs in developmental disorders. Clearly, important differences exist in the symptoms of self-injury in different conditions. Similarly, it is possible that SIB has an entirely different functional role in these different disorders (Baron-Cohen 1989). Thus, it may be argued that even if a single agent is useful in various conditions, its effects depend on different psychobiologic mechanisms. A particularly important integrative perspective may be that of evolutionary psychology, which may shed light on the adaptive function of stereotypic behavior (Stein et al. 1994a). Ultimately, an integration of biologic, psychologic, and cultural data is needed in the study of SIBs (Favazza 1987).

# References

American Psychiatric Association: Diagnostic and Statistical Manual of Mental Disorders, 4th Edition. Washington, DC, American Psychiatric Association, 1994

Anderson GM, Freedman DX, Cohen DJ, et al: Whole blood serotonin in autistic and normal subjects. J Child Psychol Psychiatr 28:885–900, 1987

Anderson LT, Campbell M, Adams P, et al: The effects of haloperidol on discrimination learning and behavioral symptoms in autistic children. J Autism Dev Disord 19:227–239, 1989

Anderson LT, Ernst M: Self-injury in Lesch-Nyhan diseases. J Autism Dev Disord 24:67–81, 1994

Bailey A, Phillips W, Rutter M: Autism: toward an integration of clinical, genetic, neuropsychological, and neurobiological perspectives. J Child Psychol Psychiatry 37:89–126, 1996

Baron-Cohen S: Do autistic children have obsessions and compulsions? Br J Clin Psychol 193–200, 1989

Bauman ML: Microscopic neuroanatomic abnormalities in autism. Pediatrics 87:S791–S796, 1991

Berkson G: Repetitive stereotyped behaviors. Am J Ment Defic 88:239–246, 1983

Bodfish JM, Crawford TM, Powell SB, et al: Compulsions in adults with mental retardation: prevalence, phenomenology, and comorbidity with stereotypy and self-injury. Am J Ment Retard 100:183–192, 1995

Breese GR, Hulebak KL, Napier TC, et al: Enhanced muscimol-induced behavioral responses after 6-OHDA lesions. Psychopharmacology 91:356–362, 1967

Breese GR, Baumeister AA, McGown T, et al: Behavioral differences between neonatal and adult 6-hydroxydopamine-treated rats to dopamine agonists: relevance to neurological symptoms in clinical syndromes with reduced brain dopamine. J Pharmacol Exp Ther 231:343–354, 1984

Bryson Y, Sakati N, Nyhan WL, et al: Self-injurious behavior in the Cornelia de Lange syndrome. Am J Ment Defic 76:319–324, 1971

Campbell M, Adams P, Small AM, et al: Efficacy and safety of fenfluramine in autistic children. J Am Acad Child Adolesc Psychiatry 27:434–439, 1988

Campbell M, Anderson LT, Small AM, et al: Naltrexone in autistic children: behavioral symptoms and attentional learning. J Am Acad Child Adolesc Psychiatry 32:1283–1291, 1993

Cataldo MF, Harris J: The biological basis for self-injury in the mentally retarded. Analysis and Intervention in Developmental Disabilities 2:21–39, 1982

Chamberlain RS, Herman BH: A novel biochemical model linking dysfunctions in brain melatonin, proopiomelanocortin peptides, and serotonin in autism. Biol Psychiatry 28:773–793, 1990

Clarke DJ, Waters J, Corbett JA: Adults with Prader-Willi syndrome: abnormalities of sleep and behavior. J Royal Soc Med 82:21–24, 1989

Coccaro EF, Siever LJ, Klar HM, et al: Serotonergic studies in patients with affective and personality disorders: correlates with suicidal and impulsive aggressive behavior. Arch Gen Psychiatry 46:587–599, 1989

Cohen SA, Underwood MT: The use of clozapine in a mentally retarded and aggressive population. J Clin Psychiatry 55:440–444, 1994

Comings DE, Comings BG: Clinical and genetic relationships between autism–pervasive developmental disorder and Tourette syndrome: a study of 19 cases. Am J Med Genet 39:180–191, 1991

Cook EH: Autism: review of neurochemical investigation. Synapse 6:292–308, 1990

Cook EH Jr, Courchesne R, Lord C, et al: Evidence of linkage between the serotonin transporter and autistic disorder. Molecular Psychiatry 2:247–250, 1997

Cook EH, Rowlett R, Jaselskis C, et al: Fluoxetine treatment of children and adults with autistic disorder and mental retardation. J Am Acad Child Adolesc Psychiatry 31:739–745, 1992

Cooper SJ, Dourish CT: Neurobiology of Stereotyped Behavior. Oxford, England, Clarendon Press, 1990

Cronin GM, Wiepkema PR, Van Ree JM: Endorphins implicated in stereotypies of tethered sows. Experientia 42:198–199, 1986

Curzon G: Serotonin and appetite, in The Neuropharmacology of Serotonin. Edited by Whitaker-Azmita PM, Peroutka SJ. New York, New York Academy of Sciences, 1990

Dunn M: Neurophysiologic observations in autism and implications for neurological dysfunction, in The Neurobiology of Autism. Edited by Bauman ML, Kemper TL. Baltimore, MD, The Johns Hopkins University Press, 1994, pp 45–65

Dunnett SB, Sirinathsinghji JD, Heavens R, et al: Monoamine deficiency in a transgenic (HPRT) mouse model of Lesch-Nyhan syndrome. Brain Res 501:401–406, 1989

Ernst M, Zametkin AJ, Matochik JA, et al: Presynaptic dopaminergic deficits in Lesch-Nyhan disease. N Engl J Med 334:1568–1572, 1996

Farber JM: Psychopharmacology of self-injurious behavior in the mentally retarded. J Am Acad Child Adolesc Psychiatry 26:296–302, 1987

Favazza AR: Bodies Under Siege: Self-Mutilation and Body Modification in Culture and Psychiatry. Baltimore, MD, The Johns Hopkins University Press, 1987

Fiser RH Jr, Bray GA, Carrel RE, et al: Evidence for hypothalamic-pituitary dysfunction in the Prader-Willi syndrome. Pediatr Res 8:368, 1974

Garber HJ, McGonigle JJ, Slomka G, et al: Clomipramine treatment of stereotypic behaviors and self-injury in patients with mental disabilities. J Am Acad Child Adolesc Psychiatry 31:1157–1160, 1992

Gillessen-Kaesbach G, Robinson W, Lohmann D, et al: Genotype-phenotype correlation in a series of 167 deletion and non-deletion patients with Prader-Willi syndrome. Hum Genet 96:638–643, 1995

Goldstein M, Kuga S, Kusano N, et al: Dopamine agonist induced self-mutilative biting behavior in monkeys with unilatreal ventromedial tegmental lesions of the brainstem: possible pharmacological model for Lesch-Nyhan syndrome. Brain Res Bull 367:114–119, 1986

Gordon CT, State RC, Nelson JE, et al: A double-blind comparison of clomipramine, desipramine, and placebo in the treatment of autistic disorder. Arch Gen Psychiatry 50:441–447, 1993

Greenberg A, Coleman M: Depressed whole blood serotonin levels associated with behavioral abnormalities in the de Lange syndrome. Pediatrics 52:720–724, 1973

Greenswag LR: Adults with Prader-Willi syndrome: a survey of 232 cases. Dev Med Child Neurol 29:145–152, 1987

Gualtieri CT, Schroeder SR: Pharmacology of self-injurious behavior: preliminary test of the D1 hypothesis. Psychopharmacol Bull 25:366–71, 1989

Guess D, Carr E: Emergence and maintenance of stereotypy and self-injury. Am J Ment Retard 96:299–319, 1991

Hellings JA, Warnock JK: Self-injurious behaviour and serotonin in Prader-Willi syndrome. Psychopharmacol Bull 30:245–250, 1994

Hellings JA, Kelley LA, Gabrielli WF, et al: Sertraline response in adults with mental retardation and autistic disorder. J Clin Psychiatry 57:333–336, 1996

Herman BH: A possible role of proopiomelanocortin peptides in self-injurious behavior. Prog Neuropsychopharmacol Biol Psychiatry 145:109–139, 1990

Herman BH, Hammock MK, Egan J, et al: A role of opioid peptides in self-injurious behavior: dissociation from autonomic nervous system functioning. Dev Pharmacol Ther 12:81–89, 1989

Holm VA: The diagnosis of Prader-Willi syndrome, in Prader-Willi Syndrome. Edited by Holm VA, Sulzbacher SJ, Pipes P. Baltimore, MD, University Park Press, 1981, pp 27–44

Horwitz B, Rumsey JM: Positron emission tomography: implications for cerebral dysfunction in autism, in The Neurobiology of Autism. Edited by Bauman ML, Kemper TL. Baltimore, MD, The Johns Hopkins University Press, 1994, pp 102–118

Hoshino Y, Tachibana R, Watanabe M, et al: Serotonin metabolism and hypothalamic-pituitary function in children with infantile autism and minimal brain dysfunction. Jpn J Psychiatry Neurol 25:937–945, 1984

Jankovic J, Caskey TC, Stout T, et al: Lesch-Nyhan syndrome: a study of motor behavior and cerebrospinal fluid neurotransmitters. Ann Neurol 23:466–469, 1988

Jimerson DC, Lesem MD, Hegg AP, et al: Serotonin in human eating disorders, in The Neuropharmacology of Serotonin. Edited by Whitaker-Azmita PM, Peroutka SJ. New York, New York Academy of Sciences, 1990

Jinnah HA, Wojcik BE, Hunt M, et al: Dopamine deficiency in a genetic mouse model of Lesch-Nyhan disease. J Neurosci 14:1164–1175, 1994

Johnson HG, Ekman P, Friesen W: A behavioral phenotype in the de Lange syndrome. Pediatr Res 10:843–850, 1976

Kapur S, Remington G: Serotonin-dopamine interaction and its relevance to schizophrenia. Am J Psychiatry 153:466–476, 1996

Kastner T, Finesmith R, Walsh K: Long-term administration of valproic acid in the treatment of affective symptoms in people with mental retardation. J Clin Psychopharmacol 13:448–451, 1993

King BH: Self-injury by people with mental retardation: a compulsive behavior hypothesis. Am J Ment Retard 98:93–112, 1993

Kohen D: Eltoprazine for aggression in mental handicap. Lancet 341:628–629, 1993

Kopin IJ: Neurotransmitters and the Lesch-Nyhan syndrome. N Engl J Med 305:1148–1149, 1981

Kyriakides M, Silverstone T, Jeffcoate W, et al: Effect of naloxone on hyperphagia in Prader-Willi syndrome. Lancet 8173:876–877, 1980

Lake CR, Ziegler MG: Lesch-Nyhan syndrome: low dopamine-betahydroxylase activity and diminished sympathetic response to stress and posture. Science 196:905–906, 1977

Lapierre YD, Reesal R: Pharmacologic management of aggressivity and self-mutilation in the mentally retarded. Psychiatr Clin North Am 9:745–754, 1986

Leonard HL, Lenane MC, Swedo SE, et al: A double-blind comparison of clomipramine and desipramine treatment of severe onychophagia (nail biting). Arch Gen Psychiatry 48:821–827, 1991

Lesch M, Nyhan WL: A familial disorder of uric acid metabolism and central nervous system function. Am J Med 36:561–70, 1964

Leuba C: Toward some integration of learning theories: the concept of optimal stimulation. Psychol Rep 1:27–32, 1955

Leventhal BL, Cook EH, Morfold M, et al: Clinical and neurochemical effects of fenfluramine in children with autism. J Neuropsychiatry Clin Neurosci 5:307–315, 1993

Lewis MH, Bodfish JW, Powell SB, et al: Clomipramine treatment for self-injurious behavior in mental retardation: a double-blind comparison with placebo. Am J Retard 100:654–665, 1996

Lloyd KG, Hornykiewics O, Davidson L, et al: Biochemical evidence of dysfunction of brain neurotransmitters in th Lesch-Nyhan syndrome. N Engl J Med 305:1106–1011, 1981

Lovaas I, Newsom C, Hickman C: Self-stimulatory behavior and perceptual reinforcement. J Appl Behav Anal 20:45–68, 1987

Luchins DJ, Dojka D: Lithium and propranolol in aggression and self-injurious behavior in the mentally retarded. Psychopharmacol Bull 3:372–375, 1989

Markowitz PI: Effect of fluoxetine in self-injurious behavior in the developmentally disabled: a preliminary study. J Clin Psychopharmacol 12:27–31, 1992

Mascari MJ, Gottlieb W, Rogan PK, et al: The frequency of uniparental disomy in Prader-Willi syndrome: implications for molecular diagnosis. N Engl J Med 326:1599–1607, 1992

McBride PA, Anderson GM, Hertig ME, et al: Serotonergic responsivity in male young adults with autistic disorder: results of a pilot study. Arch Gen Psychiatry 46:213–221, 1989

McBride PA, Anderson GM, Shapiro T: Autism research: bringing together approaches to pull apart the disorder. Arch Gen Psychiatry 53:980–983, 1996

McDougle CJ, Price LH, Volkmar FR, et al: Clomipramine in autism: preliminary evidence of efficacy. J Am Acad Child Adolesc Psychiatry 31:739–745, 1992

McDougle CJ, Goodman WK, Leckman JF, et al: Haloperidol addition in flu-
    voxamine-refractory obsessive-compulsive disorder: a double-blind placebo-
    controlled study in patients with and without tics. Arch Gen Psychiatry
    51:302–308, 1994

McDougle CJ, Kresch LE, Goodman WK, et al: A case-controlled study of repetitive
    thoughts and behavior with autistic disorder and obsessive-compulsive disor-
    der. Am J Psychiatry 152:772–777, 1995

McDougle CJ, Naylor ST, Cohen DJ, et al: A double-blind, placebo-controlled
    study of fluvoxamine in adults with autistic disorder. Arch Gen Psychiatry
    53:1001–1008, 1996a

McDougle CJ, Naylor ST, Cohen DJ, et al: Effects of tryptophan depletion in
    drug-free adults with autistic disorder. Arch Gen Psychiatry 53:993–1000,
    1996b

Mikkelsen EJ: Low-dose haloperidol for stereotypic self-injurious behavior in the
    mentally retarded. N Engl J Med 315:398–399, 1986

Mikkelsen EJ, Albert LG, Emens M, et al: The efficacy of antidepressant medication
    for individuals with mental retardation. Psychiatr Ann 27:198–206, 1997

Minshew NJ: Indices of neural function in autism: clinical and biological implica-
    tions. Pediatrics 87:774–780, 1991

Mizuno T, Yugari Y: Self-mutilation in Lesch-Nyhan syndrome. Lancet 1:761, 1974

Mizuno T, Yugari Y: Prophylactic effect of L-5HTP on self-mutilation in the Lesch-
    Nyhan syndrome. Neuropadiatrie 6:13–23, 1975

Nyhan WL: Behavior in the Lesch-Nyhan syndrome. J Autism Child Schizophr
    19:79–95, 1976

Oliver C: Self-injurious behavior: from response to strategy, in Research to Prac-
    tice? Implications of Research on the Challenging Behaviour of People with
    Learning Disability. Edited by Kiernan C. Avon, England, BILD Publications,
    1983

Osman OT, Loschen EL: Self-injurious behavior in the developmentally disabled:
    pharmacologic treatment. Psychopharmacol Bull 28:439–449, 1992

Panskepp J: A neurochemical theory of autism. Trends Neurosci 2:174–177, 1979

Perry R, Campbell M, Adams P, et al: Long-term efficacy of haloperidol in autistic
    children: continuous versus discontinuous administration. J Am Acad Child
    Adolesc Psychiatry 28:87–92, 1989

Pies RW, Popli AP: Self-injurious behavior: pathophysiology and implications for
    treatment. J Clin Psychiatry 56:580–588, 1995

Prader A, Labhart A, Willi H: Ein syndrom von adipositas, kleinwuchs, kryp-
    tochismus und oligophrenie nach myatonieartigem zustand im neuge-
    borenenalter. Schweizerische Medizinische Wochenschrift 86:1260–1261, 1956

Rapin I: Autism. N Engl J Med 337:97–104, 1997

Ratey JJ, Lindem KJ: β-Blockers as primary treatment for aggression and self-injury
    in the developmentally disabled, in Mental Retardation: Developing Pharma-
    cotherapies. Edited by Ratey JJ. Washington, DC, American Psychiatric Press,
    1991, pp 51–81

Ratey JJ, Sovner R, Mikkelsen E, et al: Buspirone therapy for maladaptive behavior and anxiety in developmentally disabled persons. J Clin Psychiatry 50:382–384, 1989

Ricketts RW, Goza AB, Ellis CR, et al: Fluoxetine treatment of severe self-injury in young adults with mental retardation. J Am Acad Child Adolesc Psychiatry 32:865–869, 1993

Ricketts RW, Goza AB, Ellis CR, et al: Clinical effects of buspirone on intractable self-injury in adults with mental retardation. J Am Acad Child Adolesc Psychiatry 33:270–276, 1994

Ridley RM: The psychology of perseverative and stereotyped behavior. Prog Neurobiol 44:221–231, 1994

Rothenberger A: Psychopharmacological treatment of self-injurious behavior in autism. Acta Paedopsychiatr 56:99–104, 1993

Rubin M: Use of atypical antipsychotics in children with mental retardation, autism, and other developmental disabilities. Psychiatr Ann 27:219–221, 1997

Sanchez LE, Campbell M, Small AM, et al: A pilot study of clomipramine in young autistic children. J Am Acad Child Adolesc Psychiatry 35:537–544, 1996

Sandman CA: β-Endorphin dysregulation in autistic and self-injurious behavior: a neurodevelopmental hypothesis. Synapse 2:193–199, 1988

Sandman CA: The opiate hypothesis in autism and self-injury. J Child Adolesc Psychopharmacol 1:237–248, 1990

Schepis C, Failla P, Siragusa M, et al: Skin-picking: the best cutaneous feature in the recognition of Prader-Willi syndrome. Int J Dermatol 33:866–867, 1994

Selikowitz M, Sunman J, Pendergast A, et al: Fenfluramine in Prader-Willi syndrome: a double-blind, placebo controlled trial. Arch Dis Childhood 65:112–114, 1990

Shear CS, Nyhan WL, Kirman BH, et al: Self-mutilative behavior as a feature of the de Lange syndrome. J Pediatrics 78:506–509, 1971

Silverstein FS, Johnston MV, Hutchinson RJ, et al: Lesch-Nyhan syndrome: CSF neurotransmitter abnormalities. Neurology 35:907–911, 1985

Singh NN, Pulman RM: Self-injury in the de Lange syndrome. J Ment Defic Res 23:79–84, 1979

Stein DJ: The neurobiology of obsessive-compulsive disorder. The Neuroscientist 2:300–305, 1996

Stein DJ, Hollander E: Dermatology and conditions related to obsessive-compulsive disorder. J Am Acad Dermatol 26:237–242, 1992

Stein DJ, Hollander E, Liebowitz MR: Neurobiology of impulsivity and impulse control disorders. J Neuropsych Clin Neurosci 5:9–17, 1993

Stein DJ, Dodman NH, Borchelt P, et al: Behavioral disorders in veterinary practice: relevance to psychiatry. Compr Psychiatry 35:275–285, 1994a

Stein DJ, Keating J, Zar HJ, et al: A survey of the phenomenology and pharmacotherapy of compulsive and impulsive-aggressive symptoms in Prader-Willi syndrome. J Neuropsych Clin Neurosci 6:23–29, 1994b

Stern LM, Walker MK, Sawyer MG, et al: A controlled crossover trial of fenfluramine in autism. J Child Psychol Psychiatry 31:569–585, 1990

Stout RJ: Fluoxetine for the treatment of compulsive facial picking. Am J Psychiatry 147:370, 1990

Swedo SE, Leonard HL, Rapoport JL, et al: A double-blind comparison of clomipramine and desipramine in the treatment of trichotillomania (hair pulling). N Engl J Med 321:497–501, 1989

Taylor DV, Rush D, Hetrick WP, et al: Self-injurious behavior within the menstrual cycle of women with mental retardation. Am J Ment Retard 97:659–64, 1993

Tiihonen J, Hakola P, Paanila J, et al: Eltoprazine for aggression in schizophrenia and mental retardation. Lancet 341:307, 1993

Van Praag HM, Plutchik R, Conte H: The serotonin hypothesis of (auto)aggression. Ann N Y Acad Sci 487:150–167, 1986

Verhoeven WMA, Tuinier S, Sijben NAS, et al: Eltoprazine in mentally retarded self-injuring patients behaviors. Lancet 340:1037–1038, 1992

Warnock JK, Kestenbaum T: Pharmacologic treatment of severe skin-picking behaviors in Prader-Willi syndrome: two case reports. Arch Dermatol 128:1623–1625, 1992

Watts RW, Spellacy E, Gibbs DA, et al: Clinical, post-mortem, biochemical and therapeutic observations on the Lesch-Nyhan syndrome with particular reference to the neurological manifestations. Q J Med 51:43–78, 1982

Wickham EA, Reed JV: Lithium for the control of aggressive and self-mutilating behavior. Int Clin Psychopharmacol 2:181–190, 1987

Willemsen-Swinkels SH, Buitelaar JK, Nijhof GJ, et al: Failure of naltrexone hydrochloride to reduce self-injurious and autistic behavior in mentally retarded adults: double-blind placebo-controlled studies. Arch Gen Psychiatry 52:766–773, 1995

Winchel RM, Stanley M: Self-injurious behavior: a review of the behavior and biology of self-mutilation. Am J Psychiatry 148:306–317, 1991

Wong DF, Harris JC, Naidu S, et al: Dopamine transporters are markedly reduced in Lesch-Nyhan disease in vivo. Proc Natl Acad Sci USA 93:5539–5543, 1996

Zlotkin SH, Fettes IM, Stallings VA: The effects of naltrexone, an oral beta-endorphin antagonist in children with the Prader-Willi syndrome. J Clin Endocrinol Metab 63:1229–1232, 1986

Zohar J, Insel TR: Obsessive-compulsive disorder: psychobiological approaches to diagnosis, treatment, and pathophysiology. Biol Psychiatry 22:667–687, 1987

Zuddas A, Ledda MG, Fratta A, et al: Clinical effects of clozapine on autistic disorder. Am J Psychiatry 153:738, 1996

# CHAPTER 3

# Psychotic Self-Injurious Behaviors
## *Phenomenology, Neurobiology, and Treatment*

Robert Grossman, M.D.

## Introduction

Some of the most severe and life-threatening self-injurious behavior (SIB) occurs among individuals with psychosis. Appropriate treatment of SIB is facilitated by a multidimensional approach. This chapter begins with an overview of the neuroanatomy and neurobiology of sensory information processing as a background for later discussion of neurobiologic studies and psychopharmacologic treatments. Phenomenology of major SIB in psychotic individuals is discussed in addition to psychosocial aspects of management.

## Sensory Pathways for Noxious Stimuli

Specific receptors exist in the body for detection of noxious stimuli. These nociceptors (*noceo* is Latin for "to injure or hurt") perform the invaluable function of signaling to the organism when potentially damaging events may be occurring. Individuals with the medical disorder of congenital insensitivity to pain are at much greater risk of sustaining severe injuries because they cannot sense the pain that warns of growing infection or worsening tissue trauma (Sternbach 1963, 1968). It has been stated that "pain is what keeps most of us from injury" (Sternbach 1968). Nociceptors are nerve endings with specialized functions that confer on them selective sensitivity to various stimuli such as pressure, heat, or local chemical milieu. Stimulation of nociceptors leads to their depolarization and the creation of an action potential in the neuron, which travels centrally to the brain via A (and C) fibers (Jessell and Kelly 1990).

Depolarization of nociceptors can occur through both direct and indirect means. Pressure (blunt or sharp tissue injury) or temperature act directly, whereas various agents associated with tissue damage or infection lead to indirect activation (depolarization). Such agents include potassium, adenosine triphosphate, and acetylcholine (all released from damaged cells), serotonin (platelets), histamine (mast cells), and others (Fields 1987). Other agents released during infection and cellular damage, such as prostaglandins, leukotrienes, and substance P, serve to sensitize nociceptors and lower their threshold for depolarization; this relates to the common experience of increased pain sensitivity in areas of tissue injury or inflammation (La Motte 1984).

Cell bodies of all neurons carrying noxious stimuli from peripheral areas are located in the dorsal root ganglia. The nociceptive fibers then enter the spinal cord, where they bifurcate, travel up and down the cord for varying lengths, and directly or indirectly connect with three major classes of neurons. Projection neurons relay incoming sensory stimulation to the brain; local excitatory and inhibitory interneurons both relay and regulate the flow of sensory information to the brain (Ruda et al. 1986). The regulatory function of these interneurons and other central nervous system regions is important, may relate to specific deficits of pain perception in psychotic individuals, and clearly results in not all stimuli reaching central areas.

Noxious stimuli are primarily transmitted contralaterally to the brain via anterolateral pathways made up of the spinothalamic, spinoreticular, and spinomesencephalic tracts. The true complexity of this system is beyond the scope of this chapter, but of key importance are synapses formed in the thalamus and the periaqueductal gray matter. Stimulation of the periaqueductal gray matter leads to a deep analgesia. Investigators have hypothesized that the thalamus functions as a filter of signals between the sensory afferents and cortex (Buchsbaum and Silverman 1968; Crosson and Hughes 1987). Additional neural pathways lead to the primary sensory cortex (located in the postcentral gyrus) and associated cortices.

A descending pain-modulatory pathway begins in the periaqueductal gray matter and terminates in the dorsal horn of the spinal cord, using both inhibitory connections with nociceptive afferents and stimulation of the aforementioned inhibitory interneurons located in this area (Jessell and Kelly 1990). Other neurons in the periventricular and periaqueductal gray area make excitatory connections in the serotonergic nucleus raphe magnus before descending, whereas noradrenergic neurons descend from the pons (Jessell and Kelly 1990).

For thousands of years, humans have been aware of the analgesic property of opiates. Only recently has it become apparent that the mechanism of opiate-induced analgesia does not occur through direct action on pain receptors in the periphery but most likely through activation of descending pain modulatory pathways. It is interesting to note that lesions of descending noradrenergic and serotonergic pathways block the analgesia of systemically administered morphine (Jessell and Kelly 1990). The origins of these descending pathways are rich in GABAergic interneurons, which are inhibitory and contain opioid receptors. Opiates such as morphine couple with these receptors and through various mechanisms lead to a decreased likelihood of neuronal depolarization and a decreased action potential duration when depolarization does occur. Therefore, the opiate is acting to decrease firing of the inhibitory interneuron, which results in a release of the inhibition or an increase in activity of the descending pathways (Yaksh and Noueihed 1985; Yaksh et al. 1980; Yoshimura and North 1983). Noradrenergic and serotonergic antidepressants, which have demonstrated their efficacy in treatment of chronic pain, may operate through activation of descending inhibitory pathways.

It is important to distinguish between nociception and pain. Nociception is the reception of signals in the central nervous system evoked by activation of nociceptors, whereas pain is a perception that involves an abstraction and elaboration of these inputs. It can be stated that nociception is more objective, whereas pain involves higher cognitive processes and is more subjective because it is under the influences of attention, anxiety, expectation, and conditioning. Pain is experienced and communicated largely through affect. As such, this is an important consideration in the study of SIB in psychotic individuals who frequently have disturbances in affective functioning.

## Phenomenology of Self-Injurious Behavior in Psychotic Individuals

### Decreased Sensitivity to Pain

Patients with schizophrenia are "less sensitive to bodily discomfort; they endure uncomfortable positions, pricks of a needle, injuries . . . burn themselves with their cigar, hurt themselves" (Kraepelin 1919, p. ??) and "even in well-oriented patients one may often observe the presence of a complete analgesia, which includes the deeper parts of the body as well as the skin. The patients . . . incur quite serious injuries, pluck out an eye, sit down on a hot stove, and receive severe gluteal burns" (Bleuler 1950, p. ?? [translation]). Kraepelin and Bleuler, respectively, made these observations close to 100 years ago. Surgeons and internists have long been aware of altered pain perception in schizophrenic individuals. In one study it was reported that pain was absent as a presenting symptom in 21% of schizophrenic inpatients with acute perforated peptic ulcer and 37% of those with acute appendicitis (Marchand et al. 1959). This finding can be compared with pain as the presenting complaint in greater than 95% of normal individuals with these disorders. Absence of pain in individuals with schizophrenia has been reported in a number of conditions, including myocardial infarction (Lieberman 1955), cancer (Talbott and Linn 1978), third-degree burns (Shattock 1950), fractures (Fishbain 1982) and postoperative pain (Marchand 1959). Mechanisms of decreased pain sensitivity may relate to altered γ-aminobuytric acid (GABA), N-methyl-D-aspartate (NMDA), and/or endogenous opioid activity and are discussed in the section on Neurobiological Considerations later in this chapter.

## Unintentional Self-Injurious Behavior in Psychotic Individuals

The focus of this book is intentional SIB, yet unintentional SIB in psychotic individuals deserves brief mention. Because pain alerts an individual to situations that require a reaction (e.g., withdrawing one's hand from a hot surface, pulling a splinter out of one's foot, limping to reduce weight bearing on an injured lower extremity, seeking medical attention), those who are less responsive to noxious stimuli are at relatively greater risk of not taking appropriate protective actions (Dworkin 1994). Unintentional SIB can produce morbidity and mortality commensurate with intentional SIB. Implications of this with regard to treatment of psychotic individuals is addressed in a later section of this chapter.

## Intentional Self-Injurious Behavior in Psychotic Individuals

Intentional SIB in psychotic individuals has been categorized by some writers as *Major SIB* (Favazza 1987). *Major* is an appropriate term because such acts are often quite astonishing in the degree of tissue damage sustained and the extent to which these behaviors clash with societal norms. The most common acts of major SIB in psychotic individuals, which are the focus of this section, are genital mutilation (transection of the penis, castration, removal of both penis and testicles) and enucleation (removal) or puncture/laceration of the eyeball. Other major SIBs that have been reported but at lesser frequencies include amputation of limbs and digits (Hall et al. 1981), removal of the tongue (Michael and Beck 1973), and even near-total removal of the face (Scheftel et al. 1986).

### Genital Self-Mutilation

Approximately 115 cases of male genital self-mutilation have been reported in English, German, and Japanese literature since the end of the nineteenth century (Greilscheimer and Groves 1979; Martin and Gattaz 1991; Nakaya 1996). Major genital mutilation in females is less common than in males, with fewer than 10 reported cases in the literature (Coons et al. 1986; Muluka 1986). In males, the most frequent genital damage appears to be equally divided between transection of the penis (approximately 25% of cases) and removal of both testicles (approximately 25% of cases). Therefore, 50% of genital SIB in males involves one of these presentations. In approximately 10%–15% of all reported major genital SIBs, the individual completely amputated his genitals—that is, penile transection along with testicular removal (Greilscheimer and Groves 1979).

Psychotic individuals, primarily those with schizophrenia but also those with affective psychoses such as depression with psychotic features and psychotic mania, make up the majority (approximately 80%) of genital mutilators (Greilscheimer and Groves 1979; Martin and Gattaz 1991; Nakaya 1996; Shore 1979). Most of these individuals state that the act was accompanied by little or no pain (Bach-Y-Rita 1974; Shore et al. 1978). It should be noted, however, that not all individuals engaging in major genital SIB are psychotic. Individuals appear to be divisible into five generalized groups: 1) young acutely psychotic males, 2) violence-prone males during alcohol intoxication, 3) males with gender identity disorder, 4) older males with psychotic depression and somatic illness, 5) and individuals with severe personality disorders acting out rageful feelings (Greilscheimer and Groves 1979; Martin and Gattaz 1991; Nakaya 1996). In contrast with the frequently impulsive nature of the act, males with gender identity disorder who may be denied or unable to afford gender reassignment surgery will often study and carefully plan their attempts at "autosurgery" (Greilscheimer and Groves 1979; Nakaya 1996; Schneider et al. 1965). Although controlled studies are lacking, literature reviews have sought to find risk factors for these behaviors (Martin and Gattaz 1991; Nakaya 1996; Sweeny and Zamecnik 1981), but because of the uncontrolled nature of these findings, these should not be regarded as scientifically validated "predictors" of genital self-mutilation (see Table 3–1).

**Table 3–1.** Potential risk factors for major genital self-mutilation in psychotic individuals

Previous history of self-mutilation

Delusions or preoccupation with sin and/or guilt, usually of a sexual nature

Religious delusions

Command auditory hallucinations instructing such behavior

Self-induced dramatic changes in physical appearance

Disturbance in sexual identity

Early loss of father or severe childhood deprivation

Perhaps the most frequent scenario is that of the psychotic male experiencing sexual urges or thoughts that are perceived as wrong, evil, or sinful. In a concrete manner of thought typical of psychotic individuals, the genitals are seen as the cause of these experiences, and therefore removing or damaging them is a quasi-logical action. Often these persons describe feelings of relief immediately after these sacrificial acts. In one report, religious psychotic experiences were noted in 34% of psychotic major self-mutilators (Nakaya 1996). Literal interpretation of Biblical passages such as Matthew 19:12 are cited by a significant number of individuals: "There are eunuchs born that way from their mother's womb, there are eunuchs made so by men and there are eunuchs who have made themselves that way for the sake of the Kingdom of Heaven." Another occurrence that may precede major genital SIB is self-induced dramatic change in physical appearance such as shaving one's head, dramatically changing one's style of clothing, or wearing flashy jewelry or make-up (Sweeny and Zamecnik 1981).

### Ocular Self-Mutilation

Retrospective literature reviews of the approximately 90 cases of major optic SIB have found that more than 75% of individuals who engage in this behavior are psychotic at the time of the event (Clark 1981; Kennedy and Feldman 1994; Witherspoon et al. 1989). The remaining cases comprise individuals with a depressive disorder, Munchausen syndrome, substance abuse, or obsessive-compulsive disorder (Kennedy and Feldman 1994). Approximately 75% of the documented cases occur in men, with an average age of 31 years (Kennedy and Feldman 1994). The most common injury is enucleation of the right eye. Patients who enucleated one or both eyes accounted for 35.5% of the subjects in one study reviewing 45 cases of intentional self-inflicted eye injuries (Kennedy and Feldman 1994). Other self-inflicted eye injuries were found to occur with the following frequencies: gouging with fingernails, 15.6%; use of a sharp instrument, 15.6%; use of pressure, 13.3%; dousing with caustic materials, 11.1%; and miscellaneous, 8.8% (Kennedy and Feldman 1994). As with genital SIB, pain is often described as absent or minimal during these events.

In two published reviews of ocular SIB, religious ideation occurred in approximately 45% of cases and sexual ideation occurred in approximately 23% of cases (Kennedy and Feldman 1994; Witherspoon et al. 1989). Risk factors for major ocular SIB are essentially the same as for major gender SIB as presented in Table 3–1 except for the last two factors.

Perhaps the most well-known example of an individual who engaged in major ocular SIB as a response to guilt is that of Oedipus, who gouged out his eyes with his mother's brooch after discovering that he had murdered his father and married his mother. The patron saints of ophthalmology—St. Medana, St. Lucia, and St. Triuana—all used self-blinding as a punishment for sinful thought. In one study, 50% of psychotic individuals who enucleated one or more eyes quoted Biblical texts as influences. Matthew 5:29 states "And if thy right eye offend thee, pluck it out." Again, primary process symbolic thought in psychotic individuals quickly focuses on the eye as the portal through which all the overwhelming and tempting stimuli of the world enter. The impairment or complete destruction of vision that results with major ocular SIB literally blinds the individual to such "temptations."

## Studies of Pain Sensitivity and Nociception in Psychotic Individuals

As the previous two sections indicated, the vast majority of people who engage in major SIBs are psychotic, with the most frequent diagnosis being schizophrenia. Most of these individuals also experience little or no pain during these behaviors. These findings suggest that investigation of nociception/pain sensitivity in psychotic subjects may aid in the understanding and treatment of these extreme and life-threatening behaviors.

Scientifically well-controlled studies in the area of pain insensitivity in schizophrenic subjects are lacking. Most of the experimental work in this area occurred before 1980, around the time when interest in endogenous opiates and opiate receptors was high. A large number of studies involving experimentally induced pain in schizophrenic subjects reported a reduced sensitivity to pain. Various painful stimuli tested included thermal pain (E.M. Kane et al. 1971; Malmo et al. 1951); cold-pressor pain, which entails the use of ice-water baths (Albus et al. 1982; Earle and Earle 1955);

electrical pain (Buchsbaum et al. 1984; Davis et al. 1979; Watson and Jacobs 1977); pin prick and pressure (Merskey et al. 1962; Stengel et al. 1955); and imagined painful situations (Petrovich 1960). In a critical review, Dworkin (1994) pointed out several methodologic problems with these studies, such as small sample sizes, questionable diagnostic reliability, problematic control groups, lack of careful examination for medication effects, limits of the psychophysical methods used in assessing pain sensitivity, and lack of distinction between perceptual deficits and pain expression.

Dworkin (1994) also pointed out that several important questions have not been adequately addressed by these studies, including whether pain insensitivity in schizophrenia varies according to the type of painful stimulus; whether certain patients with schizophrenia are more likely to have decreased pain sensitivity than others; and most importantly whether pain insensitivity in schizophrenia reflects sensory versus affective deficits. Additionally, history of SIB was often not recorded, therefore making it impossible to address whether decreased pain sensitivity existed a priori and perhaps is a risk factor for major SIB or whether SIB itself may decrease pain sensitivity. As discussed previously, pain is a subjective experience and any experiment assessing pain sensitivity relies on the subject's reported experience of the aversive stimuli. Affective processes color one's experience, and the affective flattening accompanying schizophrenia challenges the researcher to distinguish sensory from affective components contributing to decreased pain sensitivity in schizophrenia.

There appears to be only one methodologic approach adequate for measuring sensory and emotional aspects of pain insensitivity in schizophrenia. This approach is based on signal detection theory (SDT), which is also referred to as sensory decision theory or statistical decision theory. SDT provides a subject with stimuli of varying intensities and provides two useful measures. The subject is asked to indicate when and the extent to which an experience is painful. This yields one measure of response criterion that relates to the subject's affective response to the stimuli. The second measure tested is the subject's ability to discriminate between stimuli of various intensity levels. This index of sensory discriminatory ability is related to functioning of the neurosensory system (Green and Swets 1966). SDT techniques offer much but have been criticized with regard to interpretation, and response criteria can still be affected by conceptual, judgmental, motivational, emotional, and sociocultural factors (Chapman 1977, 1980).

Only one published report on pain insensitivity in schizophrenia used SDT (Dworkin et al. 1993). This study found that patients with schizophrenia had significantly poorer sensory discrimination of painful thermal stimuli than did normal control subjects and patients with mood disorders. Surprisingly, no difference was found between schizophrenic and other subjects' response criterion for reports of pain. However, among the schizophrenic subjects, a decreasing tendency to report an experience as painful was associated with greater affective flattening, fewer positive symptoms, and poorer premorbid adjustment. Dworkin (1994) interpreted these results to suggest that pain insensitivity in schizophrenia may reflect both affective and sensory abnormalities.

Other methods of assessing pain insensitivity in schizophrenia that would allow neurosensory components to be disentangled from emotional components have not been used but are technologically possible at this time. Functional imaging techniques such as positron-emission tomography (PET) and functional magnetic resonance imaging (fMRI) could be used to assess the extent to which stimuli reach higher cortical areas and how they are processed. Magnetoencephalography (MEG), which can be used to create topographic mapping of brain neuromagnetic fields in response to noxious stimuli, could also be useful in this endeavor. The measurement of brain evoked potentials in the sensory cortex in response to various painful stimuli has been studied in schizophrenia and has been found to show lower mean amplitudes and lower amplitude/intensity slopes as compared with those found in control subjects (Davis et al. 1979).

## Neurobiologic and Neuroanatomic Considerations

From even the greatly simplified discussion of the neurobiology and neuroanatomy of nociception and the caveats with regard to affective aspects of pain, it should be evident that neurobiologic study of pain insensitivity in psychotic subjects such as those with schizophrenia is extremely complex. Factors introducing high levels of complexity include multiple nociceptor types and afferent fibers, multiple activating/sensitizing substances/conditions, multiple ascending pathways, multiple ascending connections, descending inhibition at virtually every ascending connection, multiple primary messengers, multiple inhibitor receptor types, and multiple secondary messengers/intracellular mechanisms as well as the subjective elements of pain reporting and the multiple factors influencing perception of pain.

When the endogenous opiates and opiate receptor subtypes were first being characterized, it was clear that these molecules were intimately involved both in analgesia and in mood. Hypotheses about an excess of endorphins (an endogenous opiate) in schizophrenia were forwarded, but research findings addressing these hypotheses have been mixed and generally nonconfirmatory (Meltzer 1987; Mueser and Dysken 1983). Various studies suggest glutaminergic dysregulation in schizophrenia (Hirsch et al. 1997; Hoffman and McGlashan 1997), and NMDA receptor antagonists have analgesic properties (Woolf and Thompson 1991). Other interesting findings in schizophrenia research that may relate to altered pain perception include decreased cortical expression of glutamic acid decarboxylase (Akbarian et al. 1995), which is necessary for GABA synthesis. GABA plays a key role in the function of inhibitory interneurons that serve to decrease extraneous signals and increase the "signal-to-noise ratio" in the sensory system. Noxious stimuli may get lost in a system that is overstimulated and more chaotic in general. The occurrence of major SIB primarily during acute psychotic episodes may support this.

The role of the thalamus in regulating sensory input traveling to higher levels of the brain has been discussed from a structural perspective. The sensory gateway functions of the thalamus may be abnormal in schizophrenia. Many neuropathologic studies have shown anatomic change in various areas of the thalamus in schizophrenic subjects (Shapiro 1993), including decreased neuronal density (Pakkenberg 1990). Quantitative MRI studies have shown reduced hippocampal size in subjects with schizophrenia (Andreasen et al. 1994). PET scanning with coregistered MRI has revealed diminished thalamic metabolic rate and loss of normal metabolic activity patterns in schizophrenic subjects who have never received medication (Buchsbaum et al. 1996). It could not be determined whether this reduction in metabolic activity was caused by changes in excitatory, inhibitory, afferent, or efferent neuronal activity.

## Assessment of Patients Who May Be at Risk for Major Self-Injurious Behavior

The astute clinician must take several factors into account when evaluating potential risk for major SIB in psychotic patients. It should be clearly acknowledged that accurate prediction of major SIB is not possible but that certain factors should heighten the clinician's level of concern with regard to the probability of such behavior occurring. In general, as positive symptoms of psychosis increase, so does the risk of major SIB.

A thorough history is critical. Particular attention should be paid to any history of major SIB episodes and to current SIB urges. Also important is an exploration of the patient's belief systems, whether delusional or otherwise. Themes of guilt and sinfulness, especially those related to issues of sex and sexuality, deserve close attention. Presence of command hallucinations should be aggressively pursued. Clinicians should assess the degree to which patients view these experiences as symptoms of an illness and the extent to which they are able to resist the commands. Individuals experiencing hallucinations or delusions they perceive as coming from a god or other benevolent force may present as a greater risk. The ego-syntonic nature of their experience may result in family members or clinicians having greater difficulties in detecting these alterations in thought and/or perception. Additionally, an ego-syntonic or even ecstatic experience would be expected to be met with much less resistance, including decreased attempts at critical thought or reality testing. Individuals who have bipolar disorder with psychotic features, schizophrenia with marked positive as opposed to negative symptoms, or schizoaffective disorder (manic type) may be more likely to fit this picture.

## A Multimodal Approach to the Care of the Psychotic Patient Who Presents with Major Self-Injurious Behavior

The patient admitted to the hospital after performing an act of major SIB, whether admitted to a general medical unit or specialized psychiatric unit, requires an integrated multidisciplinary approach. The first priorities are the patient's medical care and working with staff reactions to facilitate the delivery of optimal treatment. Patients who have just committed major SIB are usually extremely psychotic and think their action was appropriate. They are at risk for additional major SIB and require close monitoring, at times with sedation and/or physical restraint. Psychopharmacologic treatment is discussed in the following section. Not surprisingly, staff reactions to major SIB are usually a mixture of disgust, guilt, fear, anger, hopelessness, and titillation. In the case of a psychotic individual who has transected his penis, staff may question the appropriateness of reconstructive surgery to connect the severed portion. Modern surgical techniques allow the vast majority of such cases to regain normal physiologic function after surgery. Statements such as "he didn't want it anyway" or "most of these patients kill themselves eventually" need to be addressed. Most of these patients do not view their behavior as an attempt at killing themselves but the opposite—an attempt to "save" themselves or decrease the intensity of overwhelming stimuli.

Many authors have pointed out the ambivalence that often surrounds such acts and how a significant number of patients bring their severed genitals with them when reporting what they have done. Some individuals dispose of the severed body part such as by flushing it down the toilet, whereas others may have swallowed it (Greilsheimer and Groves 1979). Most individuals usually regret what damage they have done once their acute psychosis is treated. By no means do most of the patients who have engaged in major SIB eventually kill themselves. Psychiatrists may often find themselves in the position of consulting for surgical services to which such patients have been admitted. In virtually all cases, the decision to proceed with the usual reconstructive procedure should be fully supported. Some surgeons may balk at correcting something that a person did "intentionally." It is important to point out that most of these individuals can be successfully treated and that when no longer psychotic they often regret their mutilatory actions.

Not infrequently, patients who have committed an act of major SIB are treated quite differently by staff. Staff members who otherwise act appropriately may alter their interactions, usually in decreased contact with the patient, because of their own feelings of disgust, fear, and helplessness. Staff meetings addressing such reactions toward self-injuring patients can be of great benefit, and staff members should be educated about the efficacy of pharmacologic treatment and supportive psychotherapy. Other staff reactions may include voyeuristic viewing of the patient by team members and even persons uninvolved in the patient's care.

Family members of the patient have similar negative reactions, and major SIB can further isolate psychotic individuals from the few caregivers to whom they have access. Family members should be met with, especially once the acute psychosis begins to diminish and discharge planning comes into consideration.

Psychotherapy with the patient should combine several elements. Often, the extreme feelings of guilt or sinfulness that prompt psychotic individuals to engage in an act of SIB can be mitigated through discussion of their sexual feelings and normalizing them. Clergy members can be of great assistance by meeting with the patient and helping to moderate the extremity of their views and behaviors. The key element in interactions involving the patient is that they be in a mental state that is not wholly composed of delusional thinking and hallucinatory experience.

An overall consideration for those who provide health care for chronically psychotic individuals is the patients' decreased sensitivity to pain. Complaints of pain in a psychotic individual must be taken very seriously. Similar to diabetic patients with peripheral neuropathy, chronically psychotic or schizophrenic patients can be taught to examine themselves for injuries, and physicians seeing such individuals need to both teach and practice such procedures.

## Psychopharmacologic Treatment of the Psychotic Patient with Self-Injurious Behavior

The essential principles in the pharmacologic treatment of major SIB in psychotic individuals are rapid treatment of the psychosis, establishment of a medication regimen that optimizes compliance, and sedation during acute periods of agitation. No controlled studies are available of medication use for the treatment of major SIB in psychotic individuals. Treatment recommendations are based on established clinical practices for treatment of the underlying disorder and manifesting behaviors (Table 3–2).

Most patients who engage in major SIBs meet DSM-IV (American Psychiatric Association 1994) diagnostic criteria for schizophrenia. Antipsychotic medications are the mainstay of treatment. A clear history should be obtained with regard to medications received, including dose, duration, and response. No medication is effective if not taken appropriately; therefore, compliance issues must be explored. Reports of the patient, family members, residence staff, medication levels, prolactin level, and history of filled prescriptions may all be informative. In situations of poor compliance, the contributing factors should be determined, including side effects, poor insight into illness, cognitive disorganization, or health care delivery system problems.

### *Antipsychotics*

Choice of antipsychotic agent should be based on usual psychopharmacologic considerations, which take into account patient age, comorbid medical conditions, other medications the patient is receiving, allergies, prior response, and adverse reactions. Aside from the role of psychoeducation and other psychosocial interactions to improve compliance, consideration should be given to depot formulations of haloperidol and fluphenazine and the availability of community outreach programs or structured treatment settings that facilitate regular dose delivery.

Newer atypical antipsychotic medications, which have greater specificity for D4 receptors combined with serotonergic antagonist properties, may be better tolerated by many patients and may carry lower risks of movement disorders and other adverse events that accompany long-term use. From a theoretical perspective, agents such as clozaril, olanzapine, and perhaps risperidol, which have greater efficacy in treatment of negative symptoms of schizophrenia, may be particularly suited for cases or prevention of unintentional SIB. This is based on the suggestion that decreased pain sensitivity in schizophrenia is associated with affective flattening (Dworkin 1994). Perhaps a medication more likely to bring about improve-

**Table 3–2.** Pharmacotherapy of patients with major self-injurious behavior

| Medication | Target symptoms associated with self-injurious behavior | Remarks |
|---|---|---|
| Antipsychotics | Psychosis, aggression, anxiety, ego disintegration secondary to sensory overload | Antipsychotics are first-line in major SIB. Consider atypical agents because of better side effect profile and patient compliance. Clozapine, olanzapine, and quetiapine may show higher efficacy in treatment-resistant patients but are not available as injectibles. |
| Mood stabilizers | Mania, mood lability, impulsivity, agitation | A proportion of patients with major SIB may be diagnosed as schizoaffective. In psychotic bipolar patients, divalproex loading augmented with lorazepam is as effective as an antipsychotic. Carbamazepine has a risk of aplastic anemia. Gabapentin has a sedative effect but may be less efficacious when used alone. Lithium is more poorly tolerated, fatal in overdose and lowers the seizure threshold—a greater concern in the presence of organicity. |
| Antidepressants | Impulsivity, depression, anxiety, irritability | Use if there is a significant component of depression. May cause iatrogenic mania. Selective serotonin reuptake inhibitors (SSRIs) may cause akathisia and increased agitation in psychotic patients. Combinations of SSRIs with risperidone may be associated with particularly increased akathisia. |

**Table 3–2.** Pharmacotherapy of patients with major self-injurious behavior (*continued*)

| Medication | Target symptoms associated with self-injurious behavior | Remarks |
|---|---|---|
| Benzodiazepines | Overwhelming anxiety, irritability, agitation | Most useful acutely to control anxiety and agitation. May be used until antipsychotics or mood stabilizers become effective. May result in tolerance and escalating doses if used chronically. Relatively contraindicated with current or past substance abuse. Longer-acting agents (clonazepam) are preferable. Dosing is standing or as needed. Disinhibition with increased impulsivity/aggression may occur, especially with shorter-acting agents. |
| β-Blockers | Impulsivity, aggression, dissociation, hyperarousal | Both antagonists and partial agonists may be used. Most effective in generalized, outwardly directed aggression/hostility. Propranolol most likely to cause orthostasis. All may cause depression. |

ment in affective functioning would have a parallel effect on pain sensitivity, although this speculation has not been tested to date. Unfortunately, these newer agents are not available in long-acting depot preparations.

Another consideration with regard to the newer antipsychotic agents clozaril (J. Kane et al. 1988) and olanzapine (Beasley 1997) is their greater efficacy as compared with conventional neuroleptics, which translates into higher treatment response rates in neuroleptic-resistant patients. Additionally, clozaril has been found to be effective in bipolar patients resistant to mood stabilizers and conventional neuroleptics (Zarate et al. 1995). Again, the primary goal of psychopharmacologic treatment is the reduction and/or elimination of psychosis.

### Benzodiazepines

Most patients who commit an act of major SIB present in an acutely psychotic and agitated state. In addition to an antipsychotic agent, a benzodiazepine may be useful during the time lag between the initiation of the antipsychotic medication and the clinical response. Benzodiazepines can be given on an as-needed or standing basis. In both cases the use of longer-acting agents may be preferable.

### Mood Stabilizers

A fair number of patients presenting with major SIB will be diagnosed with schizoaffective disorder or bipolar disorder with psychotic features. In patients with schizoaffective disorder, the usual practice is to combine an antipsychotic agent with a mood stabilizer such as lithium, divalproex sodium, or carbamazepine. Newer agents such as gabapentin and lamotrigine can also be considered in cases in which the aforementioned mood stabilizers are not effective. Clozapine has demonstrated efficacy as a monotherapy in the treatment of schizoaffective disorder (Kimmel et al. 1994). There is also a strong suggestion that olanzapine, which has pharmacologic activity similar to clozaril, is effective as a monotherapy for some patients with schizoaffective disorder (Glazer 1997).

Mood-stabilizing agents are also indicated for treatment of bipolar patients with psychotic features. Conventional practice in such cases is to begin treatment with both an antipsychotic agent and a mood stabilizer. The antipsychotic agent is then gradually tapered over the following months once the psychotic aspects of the patient's manic episode abates. In some patients, the technique of rapidly loading divalproex sodium alone may decrease psychosis as rapidly as in those cases in which a neuroleptic is also used (Bowden 1996; Keck et al. 1993). The usual procedure in medically healthy adults is to give 10 mg/kg twice daily and to measure plasma valproate levels every 24 hours. In general, this procedure is well tolerated, removes risks of antipsychotic medication exposure, and allows for the use of benzodiazepines such as clonazepam or lorazepam for agitation until the divalproex sodium becomes effective.

Schizoaffective and bipolar patients are not the only diagnostic groups for which a mood stabilizer can be beneficial. From a dimensional point of view, a fair number of schizophrenic patients will have marked affective components and may be in a rather ecstatic or emotionally labile state surrounding a period of major SIB. In these cases an empirical trial of a mood stabilizer can be added to the antipsychotic agent if the response to the latter alone appears to be particularly delayed or inadequate.

### Antidepressants and Electroconvulsive Therapy

The principle diagnostic groups of psychotic individuals engaging in major SIB who may benefit from treatment with an antidepressant agent include major depression with psychotic features, bipolar depressed with psychotic features, and schizoaffective—depressed. Conventional treatment of major depression with psychotic features is the combination of an antidepressant medication with an antipsychotic medication. In cases of treatment resistance, contraindications to medical treatment, or a medical emergency such as a severely depressed patient who is withdrawn, mute, or not eating, electroconvulsive therapy (ECT) is highly effective.

Patients with bipolar depression can also benefit from ECT, but the risk of a manic switch must always be attended to. Bipolar patients, if placed on an antidepressant, should virtually always be treated with a mood stabilizer simultaneously to both decrease the chances of an iatrogenic mania and increase efficacy of the antidepressant agent. There is some indication that the antidepressant buproprion is the least likely to cause mania in a bipolar patient; tricyclics are most likely to cause mania; and selective serotonin reuptake inhibitors are approximately in between (Stoll et al. 1994).

There are some indications that the mood stabilizers divalproex sodium (Bowden 1995) and gabapentin may be more effective than lithium for treatment of depressive symptoms in bipolar disorder.

## Summary and Conclusions

Major SIBs, such as castration and enucleation, are primarily committed by psychotic individuals, most of whom meet the diagnostic criteria for schizophrenia. Sensitivity to pain appears to be decreased in schizophrenic patients, which may clearly contribute to unintentional SIBs such as staring at the sun, unawareness of physical injury, or infection. It remains unclear whether decreased pain sensitivity is a risk factor for major intentional SIB or whether major SIB leads to decreased pain sensitivity. Future challenges of research in the area of pain insensitivity in schizophrenia include the need to differentiate between neurosensory and emotional aspects of the subjective experience known as pain and to take into account the neuroanatomic and neurobiologic complexity of nociceptive pathways and higher level processing of this information.

The large number of psychotic patients engaging in major SIB will have strong feelings of guilt or sinfulness, often relating to delusions, hallucinations, and experiences of a religious and/or sexual nature. Presence of command hallucinations should be determined. Major SIB by psychotic patients is usually an attempt to decrease overwhelming stimulation and is not necessarily an attempt at suicide. Nonetheless, these behaviors can certainly be life threatening and are associated with substantial tissue damage.

Appropriate treatment of the patient with major SIB entails a multidisciplinary approach. Major SIB often stirs up strong emotional reactions in both treating staff and family members. Psychoeducation of the patient and others about the treatability of the condition and about the regret often felt by patients during their recovery and return to normal thought and perceptions is helpful in ensuring appropriate delivery of care, including reconstructive surgery. Clergy members can be of assistance in helping patients modify the severity of their beliefs and normalizing the patients' experiences of sexual thoughts, which they may view as dangerous, sick, or sinful.

The primary focus in the pharmacologic treatment of psychotic patients engaging in major SIB is treatment of the underlying psychotic condition. Most frequently the diagnosis is schizophrenia, but may also be schizoaffective disorder, bipolar disorder with psychotic features, major depression with psychotic features, or psychotic disorder not otherwise specifed. Pharmacologic treatment follows current guidelines for the underlying disorder. Accurate diagnosis is important, as is initiating treatment in a setting that ensures the patient's safety from further SIB in the surrounding time period. With regard to outpatient treatment, a structured setting that increases the chances for medication compliance and allows for continued psychotherapy and close patient monitoring is often helpful.

Despite the shocking nature of major SIB in the psychotic patient, the condition is clearly treatable. The well-trained clinician or treatment team should realize that they already possess the necessary diagnostic acumen, the ability to use a multidimensional treatment approach, and the knowledge of pharmacology that constitute the major ingredients necessary for effective treatment of this patient population.

## References

Akbarian S, Kim JJ, Potkin SG, et al: Gene expression for glutamic acid decarboxylase is reduced without loss of neurons in prefrontal cortex of schizophrenics. Arch Gen Psychiatry 52:258–266, 1995

Albus M, Ackenheil M, Engel RR, et al: Situational reactivity of autonomic functions in schizophrenic patients. Psychiatry Res 6:361–370, 1982

American Psychiatric Association: Diagnostic and Statistical Manual of Mental Disorders, 4th Edition. Washington, DC, American Psychiatric Press, 1994

Andreasen NC, Arndt S, Swayze V, et al: Thalamic abnormalities in schizophrenia visualized through magnetic resonance image averaging. Science 266:294–298, 1994

Bach-Y-Rita G: Habitual violence and self-mutilation. Am J Psychiatry 131:1018–1020, 1974

Beasley CM: Efficacy of olanzapine: an overview of pivotal clinical trials. J Clin Psychiatry 15:16–18, 1997

Bleuler E: Dementia Praecox, or the Group of Schizophrenias (translation). New York, International Universities Press, 1950

Bowden CL: Predictors of response to divalproex sodium and lithium. J Clin Psychiatry 56:25–30, 1995

Bowden CL: The efficacy of divalproex sodium and lithium in the treatment of acute mania. The Psychiatry Forum 16:1–6, 1996

Buchsbaum MS, Silverman J: Stimulus intensity control and the cortical evoked response. Psychosom Med 30:12–22, 1968

Buchsbaum MS, DeLisi LE, Holcomb HH, et al: Anteroposterior gradients in cerebral glucose use in schizophrenia and affective disorders. Arch Gen Psychiatry 41:1159–1166, 1984

Buchsbaum MS, Someya T, Teng CY, et al: PET and MRI of the thalamus in never-medicated patients with schizophrenia. Am J Psychiatry 153:191–199, 1996

Chapman CR: Sensory decision theory methods in pain research: a reply to Rollman. Pain 3:295–305, 1977

Chapman CR: Pain and perception: comparison of sensory decision theory and evoked potential methods, in Pain. Edited by Bonica JJ. New York, Raven Press, 1980, pp 111–142

Clark RA: Self-mutilation accompanying religious delusions: a case report and review. J Clin Psychiatry 42:243–245, 1981

Coons PM, Ascher-Svanum H, Bellis K: Self-amputation of the female breast. Psychosomatics 27:667–668, 1986

Crosson B, Hughes CW: Role of the thalamus in language: is it related to thought disorder? Schizophr Bull 13:605–621, 1987

Davis GC, Buchsbaum MS, van Kammen DP, et al: Analgesia to pain stimuli in schizophrenics and its reversal by naltrexone. Psychiatry Res 1:61–69, 1979

Dworkin RH: Pain insensitivity in schizophrenia: a neglected phenomenon and some implications. Schizophr Bull 20:235–248, 1994

Dworkin RH, Clark WC, Lipsitz JD, et al: Affective deficits and pain insensitivity in schizophrenia, special issue: the pain system. A multilevel model for the study of motivation and emotion. Motivation and Emotion 17:245–276, 1993

Earle A, Earle BV: The blood pressure response to pain and emotion in schizophrenia. J Nerv Ment Dis 121:132–139, 1955

Favazza A: Bodies Under Siege: Self-Mutilation in Culture and Psychiatry. Baltimore, MD, The Johns Hopkins University Press, 1987

Fields HL: Pain. New York, McGraw-Hill, 1987

Fishbain DA: Pain insensitivity in psychosis. Ann Emerg Med 11:630–632, 1982

Glazer WM: Olanzapine and the new generation of antipsychotic agents: patterns of use. J Clin Psychiatry 15:27–29, 1997

Green DM, Swets JA: Signal Detection Theory and Psychophysics. New York, John Wiley and Sons, 1966

Greilsheimer H, Groves JE: Male genital self-mutilation. Arch Gen Psychiatry 36:441–446, 1979

Hall DC, Lawson BZ, Wilson LG: Command hallucinations and self-amputation of the penis and hand during a first psychotic break. J Clin Psychiatry 42:322–324, 1981

Hirsch SR, Das I, Garey LJ, et al: A pivotal role for glutamate in the pathogenesis of schizophrenia and its cognitive dysfunction. Pharmacol Biochem Behav 56:797–802, 1997

Hoffman RE, McGlashan TH: N-methyl-D-aspartate receptor hypofunction in schizophrenia could arise from reduced cortical connectivity rather than receptor dysfunction. Arch Gen Psychiatry 54:578–580, 1997

Jessell TM, Kelly DD: Pain and analgesia, in Principles of Neural Science, 3rd Edition. Edited by Kandel ER, Schwarz JH. New York, Elsevier, 1990, pp 385–399

Kane EM, Nutter RW, Weckowicz TE: Response to cutaneous pain in mental hospital patients. J Abnorm Psychol 77:52–60, 1971

Kane J, Honigfeld G, Singer J, et al: The Clozaril Collaborative Study Group. Clozapine for the treatment-resistant schizophrenic: a double-blind comparison with chlorpromazine. Arch Gen Psychiatry 45:789–796, 1988

Keck PE Jr, McElroy SL, Tugrul KC, et al: Valproate oral loading in the treatment of acute mania. J Clin Psychiatry 54:304–308, 1993

Kennedy BL, Feldman TB: Self-inflicted eye injuries: case presentations and a literature review. Hospital and Community Psychiatry 45:470–474, 1994

Kimmel SE, Calabrese JR, Woyshville MJ, et al: Clozapine in treatment-refractory mood disorders. J Clin Psychiatry 55:91–93, 1994

Kraepelin E: Dementia Praecox and Paraphrenia. Edinburgh, Scotland, E. and S. Livingstone, 1919

La Motte RH: Can the sensitization of nociceptors account for hyperalgesia after skin injury? Hum Neurobiol 3:47–52, 1984

Lieberman AL: Painless myocardial infarction in psychotic patients. Geriatrics 10:579–580, 1955

Malmo RB, Shagass C, Smith AA: Responsiveness in chronic schizophrenia. J Personal 19:359–375, 1951

Marchand WE: Practice of surgery in a neuropsychiatric hospital. Arch Gen Surg 1:123–131, 1959

Marchand WE, Sarota B, Marble HC, et al: Occurence of painless acute surgical disorders in psychotic patients. N Engl J Med 260:580–585, 1959

Martin T, Gattaz WF: Psychiatric aspects of male genital self-mutilation. Psychopathology 24:170–178, 1991

Meltzer HY: Biological studies in schizophrenia. Schizophr Bull 13:77–111, 1987

Merskey H, Gillis A, Marszalek KS: A clinical investigation of reactions to pain. J Ment Sci 108:347–355, 1962

Michael KD, Beck R: Self-amputation of the tongue. Int J Psychoanal Psychother 1:93–99, 1973

Mueser KT, Dysken MW: Narcotic antagonists in schizophrenia: a methodological review. Schizophr Bull 9:213–225, 1983

Muluka EAP: Severe self-mutilation among Kenyan psychotics. Br J Psychiatry 149:778–780, 1986

Nakaya M: On background factors of male genital self-mutilation. Psychopathology 29:242–248, 1996

Pakkenberg B: Pronounced reduction of total neuron number in mediodorsal thalamic nucleus and nucleus accumbens in schizophrenics. Arch Gen Psychiatry 47:1023–1028, 1990

Petrovich DV: Pain apperception in chronic schizophrenics. Journal of Projective Techniques 24:21–27, 1960

Ruda MA, Bennett GJ, Dubner R: Neurochemistry and neural circuitry in the dorsal horn. Prog Brain Res 66:219–268, 1986

Scheftel S, Nathan AS, Razin AM, et al: A case of radical facial self-mutilation: an unprecedented event and its impact. Bull Menninger Clin 50:525–540, 1986

Schneider SF, Harrison SI, Siegal BL: Self-castration by a man with cyclic changes in sexuality. Psychosom Med 27:53–70, 1965

Shapiro RM: Regional neuropathology in schizophrenia. Schizophr Res 10:187–239, 1993

Shattock FM: The somatic manifestations of schizophrenia: a clinical study of their significance. J Ment Sci 96:132–142, 1950

Shore D: Self-mutilation and schizophrenia. Compr Psychiatry 20:384–387, 1979

Shore D, Anderson DJ, Cutler NR: Prediction of self-mutilation in hospitalized schizophrenics. Am J Psychiatry 135:1406–1407, 1978

Stengel E, Oldham AJ, Ehrenberg ASC: Reactions to pain in various abnormal mental states. J Ment Sci 101:52–69, 1955

Sternbach RA: Congenital insensitivity to pain: a critique. Psychol Bull 60:252–264, 1963

Sternbach RA: Pain: A Psychophysiological Analysis. New York, Academic Press, 1968

Stoll AL, Mayer PV, Kolbrener M, et al: Antidepressant-associated mania: a controlled comparison with spontaneous mania. Am J Psychiatry 151:1642–1645, 1994

Sweeny S, Zamecnik K: Predictors of self-mutilation in patients with schizophrenia. Am J Psychiatry 138:1086–1089, 1981

Talbott JA, Linn L: Reactions of schizophrenics to life-threatening disease. Psychiatr Q 50:218-227, 1978

Watson CG, Jacobs L: Pain adaptation and emotional deficit. J Clin Psychol 33:555–557, 1977

Witherspoon CD, Feist FW, Morris RE: Ocular self-mutilation. Ann Ophthalmol 21:225–259, 1989

Woolf CJ, Thompson WN: The induction and maintenance of central sensitization is dependent on N-methyl-D-aspartic acid receptor activation: implications for the treatment of post-injury pain by hypersensitivity states. Pain 44:293–299, 1991

Yaksh TL, Noueihed R: The physiology and pharmacology of spinal opiates. Annu Rev Pharmacol Toxicol 25:433–462, 1985

Yaksh TL, Jessell TM, Gamse R, et al: Intrathecal morphine inhibits substance P release from mammalian spinal cord in vivo. Nature 286:155–157, 1980

Yoshimura M, North RA: Substantia gelatinosa neurones hyperpolarized in vitro by enkephalin. Nature 305:529–530, 1983

Zarate CA, Tohen M, Banov MD, et al: Is clozapine a mood stabilizer? J Clin Psychiatry 56:108–112, 1995

# CHAPTER 4

# Compulsive Self-Injurious Behaviors
## Neurobiology and Psychopharmacology

Dan J. Stein, M.B.
Daphne Simeon, M.D.

## Introduction

The classical compulsions of obsessive-compulsive disorder (OCD) only very rarely involve self-mutilation. However, in Tourette's syndrome, a disorder characterized by tics as well as by obsessive-compulsive symptoms, self-injurious behavior (SIB) is not uncommon. Repetitive and ritualistic SIB is also seen in the putative OCD spectrum of trichotillomania (hair pulling) and in stereotypic movement disorder (SMD) with SIB (e.g., skin picking, nail biting). In this chapter we discuss the neurobiology and pharmacotherapy of this range of compulsive SIBs.

Although the term *compulsive self-injurious behaviors* does not refer to any particular DSM category, the various symptoms discussed here possibly have some phenomenologic and biologic characteristics in common. These may arguably be compared and contrasted with those of more impulsive kinds of SIBs discussed elsewhere in this volume. There is, however, a relative paucity of research on the biology of compulsive SIBs. We begin with a discussion of SIBs in Tourette's syndrome and then discuss hair pulling and other compulsive SIBs.

## Tourette's Syndrome

Compulsive SIB is only rarely seen in OCD (Primeau and Fontaine 1987). In contrast, this symptom is not uncommon in the possibly closely related disorder of Tourette's syndrome. Although a great deal is known about the neurobiology and psychopharmacology of both OCD and Tourette's syndrome, relatively little work has focused on SIB symptoms in these disorders. In this section of the chapter we briefly review work on Tourette's syndrome that may be relevant to compulsive SIB.

Tourette's syndrome is characterized by multiple motor and vocal tics, which are repetitive, involuntary, stereotyped movements or vocalizations that are often preceded by premonitory urges (Leckman et al. 1993). Onset of Tourette's syndrome occurs in early childhood. Comorbid psychopathology, including OCD and attention-deficit/hyperactivity disorder, is common. The obsessive-compulsive symptoms in Tourette's syndrome differ somewhat from those seen in OCD (Pitman et al. 1987), and to some extent there is an overlap between the phenomenology of tics and obsessive-compulsive symptoms.

SIB is seen in 13%–53% of patients with Tourette's syndrome (Robertson 1989; Robertson et al. 1989). A wide range of behaviors may be seen, particularly head banging and self-punching or self-slapping as well as lip biting, tongue biting, eye poking, and skin picking. Medical complications have included subdural hematoma and vision impairment. In a large study, such behavior was not correlated with intellectual function, but was significantly associated with severity of motor tics and with scores of hostility and obsessionality (Robertson et al. 1989). Furthermore, SIBs have been described as compulsions occurring more commonly in patients with Tourette's syndrome than in those with OCD (Pitman et al. 1987). Thus, although the neurobiology of SIB in Tourette's syndrome has not been well studied, it is possible that it overlaps with that underlying tics and compulsions.

### Neurochemistry

Several neurochemical systems have been implicated in Tourette's syndrome, most notably the dopamine system. Preclinical studies demonstrate stereotypic movements after administration of dopamine agonists (Cooper and Dourish 1990), and clinical studies document de novo production or exacerbation of tics with these agents (Goodman et al. 1990). Although cerebrospinal fluid studies of dopamine metabolites have been inconsistent (Caine 1985; Leckman et al. 1995), a postmortem study found evidence of increased striatal dopamine transporters in Tourette's syndrome (Singer et al. 1991). Functional imaging studies have confirmed greater-than-normal striatal dopamine transporter densities (Malison et al. 1995), and in monozygotic twins with Tourette's syndrome, increased caudate D2 receptor binding was associated with increased tic severity (Wolf et al. 1996). Certainly, dopamine blockers have long proven to be a mainstay of the treatment of tics and other behavioral disturbances in the syndrome (Bruun and Budman 1996; Shapiro and Shapiro 1982).

Nevertheless, other neurotransmitter systems have also been associated with mediation of symptoms. A postmortem study found decreased levels of serotonin and 5-hydroxyindoleacetic acid (5-HIAA) in subcortical brain regions. Blood tryptophan levels have been decreased in some studies of Tourette's syndrome, and cerebrospinal fluid tryptophan levels were found to be inversely related to tic severity in one study (Leckman et al. 1995), although tryptophan depletion did not exacerbate tics or obsessive-compulsive symptoms in a small sample of patients (Rasmusson et al. 1997). Although several open-label reports have been made of serotonergic antidepressant use in Tourette's syndrome, only a few controlled studies of these agents are available (Caine et al. 1979; Kurlan et al. 1993). The serotonin reuptake inhibitors may be particularly effective in reducing comorbid OCD symptoms (Eapen et al. 1996).

Interactions between the dopamine and serotonin systems are well established at the preclinical level (DeSimoni et al. 1987). Furthermore, patients with OCD and tics may require augmentation of serotonin reuptake inhibitors with dopamine blockers (McDougle et al. 1994). Conversely, addition of serotonin reuptake inhibitors to neuroleptic treatment may be useful in the treatment of patients with Tourette's syndrome (Hawkridge et al. 1996). Nevertheless, further study is needed to clarify the safety and efficacy of such combinations (Friedman 1994; Hansen-Grant et al. 1994; Horrigan and Barnhill 1994).

Noradrenergic systems may also play a role in Tourette's syndrome. Cerebrospinal fluid noradrenaline levels were increased in patients in a recent study, and neuroendocrine challenge with the $\alpha_2$-adrenergic receptor agonist clonidine revealed a blunted growth hormone response in several studies (Leckman et al. 1995). Furthermore, controlled trials of clonidine demonstrate efficacy in the treatment of this syndrome, with reduction in tics, compulsive behavior, and other target symptoms (D.J. Cohen et al. 1980). SIB has been seen after clonidine withdrawal (Dillon 1990). It seems likely that, in Tourette's syndrome, the noradrenergic, dopaminergic, and serotonergic systems have important interactions (Leckman et al. 1986).

Several studies have suggested that abnormalities of the opioid system may exist in Tourette's syndrome (Leckman et al. 1988). A patient with Tourette's syndrome and severe SIB showed decreased dynorphin in the globus pallidum at postmortem (Haber et al. 1986). However, both opioid agonists and antagonists have been reported to be useful in some cases. Indeed, McConville et al. (1994) suggested patients may show dynamic fluctuation in the functional status of opioid neurotransmission rather than simple hypoactivity or hyperactivity. Nevertheless, further controlled studies are necessary.

Tourette's syndrome is more common in men than in women, suggesting that hormonal factors may provoke or suppress symptoms according to gender (Petersen et al. 1993a). There are case reports of anabolic steroids exacerbating tics in athletes, and an androgen receptor blocker was reported to improve tics in a small number of patients with Tourette's syndrome (Peterson et al. 1994). Further controlled study of such hormonal agents seems warranted.

### Neuroanatomy

From a neuroanatomic perspective, there is strong evidence that prefrontal basal ganglia thalamic circuits are involved in OCD (Insel 1992) and there is increasing evidence that these circuits are among those that mediate Tourette's syndrome. Although neuropathologic studies are limited, some evidence for the involvement of striatal circuits in the syndrome is available (Haber et al. 1986). Interestingly, the basal ganglia are especially vulnerable to pre- and perinatal hypoxic-ischemic injury, a significant fact given that in twins with Tourette's syndrome, there is an association between lower birth weight and increased syndrome severity (Hyde and Weinberger 1995). Neuropsychologic studies have been reviewed elsewhere (Hollander et al. 1993), and in several the results seem consistent with dysfunction in frontal-subcortical circuits. Neurosurgical interruption of these circuits has been used in cases of severe Tourette's syndrome with SIB (Robertson et al. 1990).

The strongest evidence for involvement of these circuits in Tourette's syndrome emerges from brain imaging studies. Magnetic resonance imaging (MRI) studies have found reduced basal ganglia volumes (Hyde et al. 1995; Peterson et al. 1993b; Singer et al. 1993). Positron-emission tomography (PET) studies have demonstrated decreased metabolism in ventral prefrontal cortex and ventral striatum, with increased metabolism in supplementary motor, lateral premotor, and Rolandic cortices (Braun et al. 1993). Significantly, increased metabolism in orbitofrontal cortex and putamen correlated with complex behavioral and cognitive features such as SIB (Braun et al. 1995). As in OCD, further work is needed to determine whether this reflects a primary deficit or functional compensation (Insel 1992).

## Neuroimmunology

Perhaps the most unorthodox approach to the neurobiology of OCD and Tourette's syndrome in the past several years has been the work of Swedo and others on the neuroimmunology of these disorders. It turns out that patients with Sydenham's chorea commonly have OCD, that OCD and tics may be exacerbated by streptococcal infection, and that patients with OCD or tics may demonstrate increased frequency of the D8/17 lymphocyte marker of susceptibility to streptococcal complications (Swedo et al. 1997). However, little work has been done on the neuroimmunology of compulsive SIB. Nevertheless, we return to this question later in the chapter in the discussion of trichotillomania.

## Genetics

Family studies indicate that Tourette's syndrome lies on a spectrum of related tic disorders and also that a genetic relationship exists between Tourette's syndrome and OCD (Pauls et al. 1986). Despite extensive study, no specific genetic defect has so far been found for the syndrome (Leckman 1997). Nevertheless, candidate genes may ultimately include those involved in dopaminergic activity, those with steroid response elements, or those responsible for basal ganglia development (Leckman 1997).

## Pharmacotherapy

As described in the preceeding neurobiologic sections, various different classes of medications are used to treat Tourette's syndrome. These meidations have not been independently studied to examine their efficacy specifically for the SIB aspects of the syndrome, and there is no reason to assume at this point that these warrant distinct treatment.

First-line pharmacologic treatment of Tourette's syndrome consists of antipsychotic medications (Bruun and Budman 1996; Shapiro and Shapiro 1982). Both conventional neuroleptics such as haloperidol and pimozide and atypical neuroleptics such as risperidone have been shown to be efficacious, and it remains unclear what their comparative efficacy is. Serotonin reuptake inhibitors may also be beneficial, either as monotherapy or as adjuvants to neuroleptics; both clomipramine and the selective serotonin reuptake inhibitors (SSRIs) have been used in this regard, although con-

trolled data are very limited (Caine et al. 1979; Kurlan et al. 1993). Clonidine may also have some efficacy but has received little attention (Cohen
et al. 1980). Case reports of both opioid agonist and antagonist response in
Tourette's syndrome have been described, but again further study is needed (McConville et al. 1994). Finally, a role may exist for antiandrogens
(Peterson et al. 1994).

## Trichotillomania

The term *trichotillomania* was coined over a century ago to describe hair-
pulling patients (Hallopeau 1889). The diagnosis was first included in the
DSM system in its third edition, as one of the disorders of impulse control
not otherwise specified. The DSM-III-R and the DSM-IV (American Psychiatric Association 1987, 1994) include trichotillomania as a distinct disorder within the disorders of impulse control and specify that the hair
pulling must be recurrent, result in noticeable hair loss, and be associated
with clinically significant distress or functional impairment. Hair pulling
most frequently occurs from the scalp, although it can occur from a wide
range of body areas, including the eyebrows, eyelashes, beard, axillae, and
pubis (Christenson et al. 1991a; L.J. Cohen et al. 1995). Plucking may be
confined to a single patch, may involve different areas, or may cover the
entire scalp. Some patients also report pulling hair from a child or significant other. The dermatology and dermatopathology of the lesion are characteristic (Mehregan 1970; Muller 1987).

Patients with trichotillomania may demonstrate a range of other SIBs
(Christenson et al. 1991a; Simeon et al. 1997a). Although hair pulling may
lead to significant medical complications, including trichobezoar after ingestion of pulled hair (Bouwer and Stein 1998), it is perhaps more commonly associated with significant feelings of shame and low self-esteem
(Soriano et al. 1996). Indeed, both the personal and the economic costs of
this disorder may be significant (Seedat and Stein 1998).

Systematic investigation of the neurobiology and psychopharmacology of trichotillomania began in earnest after the discovery that OCD
responded selectively to serotonin reuptake inhibitors and after the possibility was raised that a range of other disorders characterized by unwanted repetitive symptoms might have overlapping phenomenologic and
neurobiologic features (Stein and Hollander 1993). Despite the relative
paucity of studies on trichotillomania, more has been published on the
neurobiology and pharmacotherapy of hair pulling than on many other
compulsive SIBs (e.g., skin picking, nail biting). In the next sections of this

chapter we discuss the neurochemistry, neuroanatomy, neuroimmuno-logy, neuropsychology, and genetics of trichotillomania as well as some interesting animal models. We draw extensively on our previous publications in this area (Simeon et al. 1997a; Stein et al. 1998b, 1998c).

## Neurochemistry

Research on the neurobiology of hair pulling was given a significant boost by a seminal trial comparing clomipramine with desipramine in the treatment of trichotillomania (Swedo et al. 1989b). Earlier work on OCD had demonstrated that the predominantly serotonergic agent clomipramine was more effective than the predominantly noradrenergic agent desipramine (Leonard et al. 1989; Zohar and Insel 1987). This finding differentiated OCD from other conditions such as depression, which responded to a range of antidepressants, and suggested that serotonin played a specific and important role in the disorder. Swedo et al. (1989a) found that, as in OCD, trichotillomania responded selectively to the serotonin reuptake inhibitor clomipramine but not to desipramine.

Nevertheless, subsequent research has not produced entirely consistent results regarding a specific role for serotonin in trichotillomania. Although the SSRIs have seemed effective for trichotillomania in several open trials, these agents have proved disappointing in controlled trials (see below). This finding contrasts markedly with work demonstrating the efficacy of the SSRIs in OCD. Furthermore, although Swedo et al. (1993) found that trichotillomania response to clomipramine may be sustained over time, other reports have indicated that initial response to serotonin reuptake inhibitors may be lost during continued treatment (Pollard et al. 1991; Stein and Hollander 1992b). Taken together, this work shows that it may be premature to overly emphasize the specific role of serotonin in trichotillomania.

A serotonin hypothesis of OCD has received some support from studies of serotonin and other neurotransmitter metabolites (Thoren et al. 1980). However, few studies of trichotillomania patients have directly assessed monoamine concentrations. Ninan et al. (1992) obtained cerebrospinal fluid samples from a small group of patients with trichotillomania and found that 5-HIAA levels did not differ from those found in normal control subjects. However, baseline cerebrospinal fluid 5-HIAA did correlate significantly with degree of response to serotonin reuptake inhibitors. This finding is redolent of some work on OCD (Thoren et al. 1980) and suggests that in both disorders response to serotonin reuptake inhibitors may be accompanied by a fall in 5-HIAA levels.

Few studies have been made of serotonergic pharmacologic challenges in trichotillomania. Stein et al. (1995, 1997a) reported that the serotonin agonist M-chlorophenylpiperazine (m-CPP), which has resulted in exacerbation of symptoms in some studies of OCD, did not lead to an increase in hair pulling in women with trichotillomania. The interpretation of these data is not straightforward; for example, although obsessions and compulsions may be present throughout the day, hair pulling in trichotillomania is often triggered only in particular settings. Furthermore, serotonergic function differs in men and women (Carlsson et al. 1985), and neuroendocrine blunting may be more commonly seen in male patients. Of some interest, however, was the finding that subjects with trichotillomania did describe an increase in feeling "high," a phenomenon that our group had also documented in an earlier study of patients with impulsive personality disorders (Hollander et al. 1994). Thus, although serotonin may play some role in hair pulling, it is possible that serotonergic mediation of OCD and trichotillomania does not entirely overlap. It may, for example, be speculated that hair pulling in trichotillomania and self-stimulatory stereotyped behaviors in patients with impulsive personality disorders (including self-mutilation) have some overlapping characteristics (Simeon et al. 1997a).

As noted earlier, increasing evidence shows that dopamine plays a role in OCD and related disorders (Goodman et al. 1990), perhaps particularly in those with a marked motoric component. Some preliminary data indicate that dopamine also plays a role in hair pulling. A recent report noted exacerbation of hair pulling from methylphenidate administration in a series of children (A. Martin et al. 1998). A similar phenomenon can be seen in adults with trichotillomania (Niehaus and Stein, unpublished data). Furthermore, preliminary open data suggest that augmentation of serotonin reuptake inhibitors with dopamine blockers may be useful in the treatment of hair pulling (Stein and Hollander 1992b; van Ameringen and Mancini 1996). The atypical neuroleptics, which have dopamine and serotonin antagonist effects, may also be effective augmenting agents in OCD and trichotillomania (Stein et al. 1997d).

The opioid system and altered pain perception have been implicated in various forms of self-mutilation (Herman 1990). In animal studies, opioid agonists may induce autoaggression, and opioid antagonists may be particularly effective in reducing self-injurious stereotypies in younger animals (Cronin et al. 1986). Indeed, it has been suggested that excessive opioid activity underlies SIBs. An alternative hypothesis emphasizes that pain associated with SIB results in release of brain endorphins and draws a parallel between such endogenous release of endorphins and addiction to an exogenous substance. However, Christenson et al. (1994) found no significant differences in either pain detection or pain tolerance thresholds between trichotillomania patients and control subjects. On the other hand, this group (Christenson et al. 1995) has suggested that the opioid blocker naltrexone may be effective in the treatment of trichotillomania, indicating that further research on the opioid system in hair pulling may be useful.

Hormonal factors are able to induce grooming in preclinical models (Traber et al. 1988), and the onset of OCD has been associated with pregnancy (Neziroglu et al. 1992). Certainly, trichotillomania is predominantly a disorder of women in the clinical setting; it frequently begins around the time of the menarche, and in some women the symptoms are exacerbated premenstrually (Christenson et al. 1991a). Nevertheless, to our knowledge no studies have directly explored hormonal mechanisms and hair pulling. Although evidence of a specific link between hair pulling and hormonal mechanisms is insufficient at present, further work in this area seems warranted.

### Neuroanatomy

The first evidence that OCD might be mediated by specific neuroanatomic circuits emerged from clinical observations of OCD symptoms in patients with neurologic disorders (such as postencephalitic parkinsonism) with basal ganglia lesions. Current conceptualizations of striatal function in terms of the development, maintenance, and selection of motoric and cognitive procedural strategies are certainly consistent with a hypothesis of striatal dysfunction in OCD. Furthermore, recent structural and functional imaging studies have confirmed the importance of corticostriatal circuits in OCD (Insel 1992). At least some studies show decreased volume of the basal ganglia, increased activity in corticostriatal circuits at rest and during symptom provocation, and decreased activity after pharmacotherapy or behavioral therapy.

In view of the serotonergic and dopaminergic innervation of the striatum (Insel 1992), a hypothesis that emphasizes a role for this region in trichotillomania and other unwanted repetitive behaviors would seem to be consistent with the neurochemical hypotheses discussed earlier. Furthermore, preclinical data indicating that the basal ganglia are a repository for species-specific motor patterns (MacClean 1978) may help explain the specificity of such clinical symptoms and the link that they often seem to have with grooming behaviors. Nevertheless, the neuroanatomy of trichotillomania is comparatively poorly researched. Only occasional reports exist of hair pulling in association with neurologic disorders, although once again basal ganglia lesions have been implicated (Rodrigo-Escalona et al.

1997; Stein et al. 1997b). A small literature on brain imaging in trichotillomania has begun to appear, however; several structural studies using MRI have been published. Stein et al. (1997c) found no differences in caudate volume between female patients with trichotillomania and control subjects. O'Sullivan et al. (1997) similarly found no difference in caudate volumes in trichotillomania patients and control subjects but did find that those with trichotillomania had reduced left putamen volumes. This finding is of interest given work demonstrating reduced left putamen volumes in Tourette's syndrome (Singer et al. 1993), another disorder that is characterized by repetitive motoric symptoms and that may lie on the OCD spectrum.

Swedo et al. (1991) found increased right and left cerebellar and right superior parietal glucose metabolic rates in trichotillomania patients compared with control subjects. This finding does not seem to support the hypothesis that orbitofrontal basal ganglia circuits are key to this disorder and differs from findings obtained in studies of OCD and Tourette's syndrome. However, patients were scanned at rest, rather than during hair pulling or during the performance of a neuropsychologic test that might have activated these structures. Swedo et al. (1991) also found that anterior cingulate and orbitofrontal metabolism correlated negatively with clomipramine response, a result they had previously found in OCD (Swedo et al. 1989a). They concluded that increased orbitofrontal metabolism may comprise a compensatory response to basal ganglia pathology in both of these disorders. Stein et al. (1998a) studied single photon emission computed tomography (SPECT) scans in patients with trichotillomania before and after pharmacotherapy with the serotonin reuptake inhibitor citalopram. During treatment, activity was reduced in the left and right inferior-posterior and other frontal areas. In nonresponders, an increase occurred in baseline left and right superior-lateral frontal areas. These data are to some extent consistent with work suggesting that trichotillomania, like OCD, is mediated by corticostriatal circuits.

## Neuroimmunology

As noted earlier, the neuroimmunology of OCD and Tourette's syndrome has recently been the focus of some seminal studies (Swedo et al. 1997). Of particular interest to research on trichotillomania, Swedo et al. (1992) reported that, as with OCD symptoms, hair pulling may relapse after streptococcal infections. In addition, Stein et al. (1997b) reported on a patient in whom hair-pulling symptoms appeared to be closely linked with Sydenham's chorea. Both choreiform symptoms and hair pulling remitted in response to treatment with penicillin. Nevertheless, no data have yet been published that establish a causal connection between *Streptococcus* or Sydenham's chorea and hair pulling. Furthermore, Niehaus and Stein (unpublished data, 1998) recently found that the D8/17 lymphocyte marker was not more frequent in patients with trichotillomania than in control subjects. It remains possible, however, that particular subtypes of trichotillomania have a specific neuroimmunologic etiology. Further research in this area is clearly warranted.

## Neuropsychology

Several studies have explored the neuropsychologic aspects of trichotillomania. In general, these have attempted to demonstrate similarities in the neuropsychology of OCD and trichotillomania and evidence of corticostriatal involvement in both of these disorders. Rettew et al. (1991) compared the results of trichotillomania patients, OCD patients, and control subjects on a neuropsychologic battery that included the Stylus Maze and the Money Road Map test. Patients with trichotillomania had significantly more errors than did control subjects on two subtests of the Stylus Maze, a test of visual-spatial memory, whereas patients with OCD differed significantly from controls on one subtest. The authors concluded that differences between trichotillomania patients and control subjects on the Stylus Maze were consistent with spatial processing difficulties in this disorder.

Keuthen et al. (1996) found group differences between trichotillomania patients and control subjects in the Odd Man Out Test, a measure of ability to maintain mental set, and on the Rey-Osterreith Complex Figures Test, an immediate-recall test of nonverbal memory. Although no group differences were found on the Rey-Osterreith Complex Figures Test copy score, a test of visuospatial function, dysfunction was found in the trichotillmania group on the Odd Man Out Test for the stimuli of shapes but not letters. The authors wondered whether this finding reflected greater difficulty in maintaining a mental set when dealing with shapes, which are less likely to be subject to verbal mediation strategies.

Coetzer and Stein (unpublished data, 1997) compared neuropsychologic functioning in female patients with trichotillomania or OCD and control subjects. Although no significant differences were found among the three groups on any of the measures studied, the combined OCD and trichotillomania group differed significantly from control subjects in accuracy and planning on the Rey-Osterreith copy score. Again, it is possible to speculate that disruption of visual-spatial coordination and sequencing tasks may reflect damage to corticostriatal pathways in these conditions.

Nevertheless, it seems that, to date, neuropsychology research findings have been too inconsistent to clearly support such a conclusion.

Women with trichotillomania did not demonstrate increased soft signs compared with control subjects (Stein et al. 1994); nevertheless, trichotillomania patients had increased evidence of visuospatial dysfunction compared with controls. Gender effects confound interpretation of this data because increased neurologic soft signs may be more frequent in men than in women with anxiety disorder and in patients with OCD. Further work therefore needs to be done if an association between increased neurologic soft signs and trichotillomania is to be excluded definitively.

### Genetics

Increasing evidence shows that genetic contributions play an important role in the pathogenesis of OCD and related disorders. A family study of OCD and Tourette's syndrome led to the hypothesis that some patients with OCD and Tourette's syndrome may be manifesting different phenotypic expressions of an underlying genotypic abnormality (Pauls et al. 1986). Most recently, preliminary evidence for the role of specific genes in mediating OCD has been published. To date, however, few studies of the genetics of trichotillomania have been performed. Nevertheless, Christenson et al. (1992) reported that 8% of 161 trichotillomania patients had first-degree relatives with the disorder. Another study failed to show elevated rates of the disorder in first-degree relatives of trichotillomania probands but did find elevated rates of OCD (Lenane et al. 1992).

### Animal Models

We noted earlier that stereotypies in animals are increased by certain neurochemical manipulations. Of at least equal interest is recent work on several veterinary models of compulsive symptoms such as hair pulling (Dodman et al. 1997). These include acral lick dermatitis in dogs, psychogenic alopecia in cats, and feather picking in birds. These problems are rather common in veterinary practice and may have bearing on current understanding of trichotillomania. Acral lick dermatitis is a condition characterized by excessive paw licking and scratching in dogs and results in the characteristic dermatitis and other sequelae, including osteomyelitis. The disorder is seen in certain breeds of large dogs, and within breeds it may be more common in particular families. The disorder has typically been hypothesized to reflect specific behavioral stressors. Nevertheless, the pharmacotherapeutic profile of acral lick dermatitis overlaps remarkably neatly with that of OCD (Rapoport et al. 1992); thus, it responds to serotonin reuptake inhibitors but fails to respond to either desipramine or fenfluramine. The disorder may also respond to opioid agents (Dodman et al. 1988).

Psychogenic alopecia, in which excessive depilation leads to bare patches, is found in cats. Again, animal behaviorists have typically conceptualized the disorder as stress related. Although not well studied pharmacologically, several reports indicate that this disorder responds to treatment with serotonin reuptake inhibitors (Hartmann 1995; Swanepoel et al. 1998). In addition, administration of a dopamine blocker has been noted to lead to a decrease in symptoms (Willemse et al. 1994).

Feather picking in birds is seen in a range of avian species. Complications include severe hemorrhage. Phenomenologically, this behavior is again closely reminiscent of trichotillomania. Veterinarians have long believed that stress and confinement play a role in this behavior. Once again, it is interesting to note that the disorder may respond to treatment with serotonin reuptake inhibitors (Grindlinger and Ramsay 1991).

Hair pulling and other forms of stereotypic and self-injurious behaviors may also be seen in primates in captivity, particularly when they are reared in isolated or other adverse conditions or kept in poor environments. Of particular interest is the finding that socially isolated primates develop striatal cellular disorganization together with stereotypic and self-injurious behaviors (L.J. Martin et al. 1991). Furthermore, in a placebo-controlled study of fluoxetine in isolation-reared primates, fluoxetine was effective in reducing such symptoms (Wessels and Stein, unpublished data, 1997).

## Psychopharmacology

As mentioned earlier, Swedo et al. (1989a) compared clomipramine with desipramine in a 10-week crossover study of trichotillomania and found clomipramine to be significantly more effective than desipramine. Later studies have investigated the use of SSRIs in the treatment of trichotillomania. Results have so far unfortunately have been equivocal. Open-label trials of SSRIs in trichotillomania have been promising, and several groups have found fluoxetine to be useful for the disorder in open trials (Koran et al. 1992; Stanley et al. 1991; Winchel et al. 1992). In similar uncontrolled studies, Christenson et al. (1998) reported promising results using fluvoxamine, and Stein et al. (1997f) found that nearly 40% of their sample of patients with trichotillomania responded to citalopram.

Unfortunately, these uncontrolled trials suffer from several methodologic limitations. For example, variability in hair pulling over time may obscure the results of short-term trials. Controlled trials of SSRIs in trichotillomania have been disappointing. Christenson et al. (1991c) were unable to document efficacy for fluoxetine in a placebo-controlled crossover trial in which patients received 6 weeks of the active agent in doses of up to 80 mg/day. Similarly, Streichenwein and Thornby (1995) did not find efficacy for fluoxetine in a placebo-controlled crossover trial in which patients received the agent for 12 weeks.

Several open-label studies of trichotillomania have focused on agents other than SSRIs, again with promising results. O'Sullivan et al. (1998) found that venlafaxine, a serotonin-noradrenaline reuptake inhibitor, may be useful. Christenson et al. (1991b, 1995) have found that trichotillomania may respond to lithium and naltrexone, agents that have not been proven useful in OCD. Clearly, controlled trials are necessary to confirm these preliminary findings.

Few studies on pharmacotherapy augmentation for trichotillomania are available. In an open-label study, Stein and Hollander (1992b) found that pimozide augmentation of a serotonin reuptake blocker was useful for six of seven patients with the disorder. This finding has been replicated by van Ameringen and Mancini (1996), and these data are reminiscent of data found for certain patients with OCD, especially those with tics (McDougle et al. 1994). Given concerns about the safety of combining SSRIs with pimozide (Friedman 1994; Hansen-Grant et al. 1994; Horrigan and Barnhill 1994) and the superior adverse event profile of the atypical neuroleptics, the possibility that these agents are also effective in augmenting SSRIs in trichotillomania (Potenza et al. 1998; Stein et al. 1997d) deserves study.

Several other issues in the pharmacotherapy of trichotillomania also require further research. Anecdotal evidence has shown that SSRIs may not be as effective over the long term for the treatment of hair pulling as they are for OCD (Pollard et al. 1991; Stein and Hollander 1992b), although other reports are more optimistic (Keuthen et al. 1998; Swedo et al. 1993). Also, although serotonin reuptake inhibitors are useful in childhood OCD (Leonard et al. 1989), demonstration of their efficacy in childhood trichotillomania needs more extensive study (Sheika et al. 1993). Finally, the comparison of pharmacotherapy, psychotherapy, and combined treatment (and assessment of their effects on brain imaging) in the disorder deserves further attention.

## Compulsive Skin Picking

Skin picking and scratching are behaviors that not uncommonly come to the attention of clinicians. The incidence of so-called neurotic excoriations in dermatology clinics has been estimated to be around 2% (Gupta et al.

1986). Medical complications of skin picking include infection and scarring. Furthermore, skin picking may be associated with significant distress and dysfunction (Simeon et al. 1997a). At times, patients with these behaviors may meet criteria for OCD (Katz et al. 1990; Stein and Hollander 1992a). However, in most patients this is not the case. Skin picking may also be seen in patients with the OCD spectrum disorders trichotillomania (Christenson et al. 1991a) and body dysmorphic disorder (Phillips and Taub 1995). The neurobiology of compulsive skin picking, including neurochemical studies and anatomic or functional imaging, is completely unknown, and therefore at present it is impossible to speculate on common neurobiologic underpinnings between skin picking and hair pulling or OCD, despite the apparently greater-than-chance prevalence of comorbidity between these disorders (Simeon 1997a).

Earlier case reports of isolated patients had suggested that serotonin reuptake inhibitors might have a role in the treatment of skin picking, both clomipramine (Gupta et al. 1986), and fluoxetine (Gupta and Gupta 1993; Stein et al. 1993; Stout 1990). Similarly, a retrospective treatment review of body dysmorphic disorder patients with skin picking indicated that serotonin reuptake inhibitors were effective in about half of 33 subjects, whereas other agents were not (Phillips and Taub 1995). In a recent open prospective trial of sertraline in 30 patients with skin picking, 68% of patients showed significant improvement. The mean daily dose for the responders was 95 mg/day, and improvement tended to occur at about 1 month's time (Kalivas et al. 1996).

Finally, in the only controlled treatment study to date, Simeon et al. (1997b) found that fluoxetine at a mean dose of 55 mg/day for 10 weeks was significantly superior to placebo in decreasing the behavior in 21 adults with chronic pathologic skin picking by some but not all of the measures used. Six of the 10 fluoxetine-assigned patients who completed the trial were all significantly improved by the last month; four of these were rated as much improved and two as very much improved. One fluoxetine subject who dropped out before the end of the study experienced significant worsening of his picking, which appared to be associated with severe fluoxetine-induced jitteriness. These results are promising but need replication with larger samples and longer duration of treatment. A controlled trial of clomipramine in compulsive skin picking would also be very desirable.

## Compulsive Nail Biting

Nail biting, or onychophagia, is a common behavior that is not, however, necessarily benign (Hadley 1984; Leonard et al. 1991). Nail biting may be associated with serious infection, nail bed damage and scarring, cranio-mandibular dysfunction, and dental disorders. The apparent ubiquity of mild nail biting should not discourage clinical and research attention to patients with more severe forms of the behavior.

In a controlled crossover treatment trial of 25 adults with severe chronic nail biting, clomipramine appeared to be more effective than desipramine, although results were not as robust as those seen in classic OCD (Leonard et al. 1991). Patients who completed the study received clomipramine for a total of 5 weeks and reached a mean dose of 120 mg/day. The positive response was modest, with a roughly 30% decrease in the severity of the behavior, and only two subjects completely stopped biting their nails. The authors emphasized that there was a very high drop-out rate at every stage of the study, which contrasted that seen in other psychiatric treatment trials. They did, however, suggest that this differential pharmacologic response pattern may be consistent with the hypothesis that similar biologic systems mediate a spectrum of grooming disorders, including OCD and trichotillomania (Leonard et al. 1991).

## Other Compulsive Self-Injurious Behaviors

Several studies have been done of various stereotypic behaviors or habits—whether self-injurious or not—in intellectually normal adults. In a self-report study of habits in 286 college students, Hansen et al. (1990) found that no one reported having no habits and that the mean number of habits reported was 6.5. The most common habits were playing with hair (70.6%), nail biting (63.6%), playing with objects, and leg shaking. However, the most problematic habits were nail biting, neck twisting, moving (e.g., clicking, grinding) teeth, and face touching. Habits were noted to have a negative impact on self-evaluation, appearance, and health. Nevertheless, none of the subjects had chosen a mental health professional as a primary source of treatment.

A range of other common self-injurious stereotypies may be seen in intellectually normal adults, including lip biting and eye rubbing (Favazza 1987). Certain kinds of stereotypies, such as thumb sucking and head banging, appear more common in children, although on occasion these behaviors may also be seen in intellectually normal adults (Stein et al. 1997e). Most importantly, stereotypic behaviors may be associated with significant medical complications, and they may also lead to distressing feelings of shame and lowered self-esteem (Joubert 1993) as well as to social avoidance and occupational impairment.

Castellanos et al. (1996) undertook clinical interviews in subjects who responded to a newspaper advertisement that specifically mentioned rocking and head banging. Of 52 potential subjects screened by telephone, 32 had been previously diagnosed with a psychiatric disorder or were otherwise excluded. Of 20 who were interviewed in person, 12 met criteria for SMD, and 8 of these had rocking or thumb sucking behaviors. In 11 of the 12 SMD subjects, onset occurred before age 7. Also, a lifetime history of a mood or anxiety disorder was present in 11 of the 12 SMD subjects. Of the 8 rockers, 4 had a first-degree relative with a history of a similar repetitive behavior.

Relatively little work has been undertaken on the neurobiology or pharmacotherapy of these kinds of symptoms in intellectually normal adults. Of some interest, our group (Niehaus et al. 2000) found that in a college population, the total number of stereotypic behaviors was significantly associated with increased scores of obsessive-compulsive symptoms, perfectionism, and impulsive-aggressive traits. In their pioneering study, Castellanos et al. (1996) compared clomipramine, a predominantly serotonergic reuptake inhibitor, and desipramine, a predominantly noradrenergic reuptake inhibitor, in a crossover trial. Although clomipramine appeared promising in several cases, too few patients completed the trial to demonstrate a clear benefit of clomipramine over desipramine.

Nevertheless, several case reports suggest that serotonin reuptake inhibitors may be useful in patients with various kinds of stereotypic SIBs (Stein and Simeon 1998; Stein et al. 1997e). A possible role for dopamine blockers, and the new atypical neuroleptics in particular, also deserves further consideration. Ultimately, controlled and long-term studies are needed to formulate rational approaches to the pharmacotherapy of these SIBs.

## Conclusion

The neurobiology of hair pulling and other compulsive SIBs in adults without obvious neuropsychiatric impairment is not very well understood; this lack of knowledge parallels our relatively limited knowledge of how best to manage these symptoms. Nevertheless, several interesting leads have emerged in recent years. There is tentative support for the hypotheses that serotonergic, dopaminergic, and opioid systems mediate compulsive symptoms such as hair pulling, and that striatal circuits, which link in turn to cortex and cerebellum, may also play a significant role.

The preclinical literature on compulsive SIBs in animals provides several interesting leads. For example, the appearance of SIB after the administration of dopamine agonists parallels some clinical findings. Similarly, findings that stereotypical and self-injurious behaviors in isolated primates are associated with basal ganglia pathology (L.J. Martin et al. 1991) and respond to serotonin reuptake inhibitors (Wessels and Stein, unpublished data, 1997) are thought provoking. De Waal (1996) has suggested that in some primates, grooming and skin picking after injury may be useful in promoting skin healing.

The extent to which the biology of different compulsive self-injurious and stereotypic behaviors overlap remains unclear. Such behaviors range from near-normal phenomena (nail biting) to severely pathologic symptoms in patients with neuropsychiatric disorders (e.g., self-mutilation in autism). Ultimately, an understanding of the neurobiology of compulsive SIB may have significant clinical implications not only for the many patients with these symptoms but also for a range of other disorders characterized by unwanted repetitive behaviors.

As with the uncertainty regarding common neurobiologic underpinnings in the range of compulsive SIBs that we have discussed, no uniform pharmacologic treatment guidelines are currently available for these various behaviors, although similarities in treatment approaches exist. In Tourette's syndrome, antipsychotics are the mainstay treatment, with serotonin reuptake inhibitors used as a common second-line or adjuvant treatment. Conversely, in compulsive hair pulling, skin picking and nail biting, serotonin reuptake inhibitors are the first-line treatment, although both open trials and controlled studies have not always been consistent about the efficacy of either clomipramine or the SSRIs in these behaviors; response appears less robust and likely than in OCD, and the maintenance of response over time is also in question. Nevertheless, trials of these medications are definitely warranted in patients with significant compulsive self-injury symptoms that lead to subjective distress or interference with functioning. Less-frequently-used medications that may be useful adjuvants include naltrexone, lithium and atypical antipsychotics.

## References

American Psychiatric Association: Diagnostic and Statistical Manual of Mental Disorders, 3rd Edition Revised. Washington, DC, American Psychiatric Association, 1987

American Psychiatric Association: Diagnostic and Statistical Manual of Mental Disorders, 4th Edition. Washington, DC, American Psychiatric Association, 1994

Bouwer C, Stein DJ: Trichobezoars in trichotillomania: case report and literature review. Psychosom Med 60:658–660, 1998

Braun AR, Stoetter B, Randolph C, et al: The functional neuroanatomy of Tourette's syndrome, an FDG-PET study, I: regional changes in cerebral glucose metabolism differentiating patients and controls. Neuropsychopharmacology 9:277–291, 1993

Braun AR, Randolph C, Stoetter B, et al: The functional neuroanatomy of Tourette's syndrome: an FDG-PET study, II: relationships between regional cerebral metabolism and associated behavioral and cognitive features of the illness. Neuropsychopharmacology 13:151–168, 1995

Bruun RD, Budman CL: Risperidone as a treatment for Tourette's syndrome. J Clin Psychiatry 57:29–31, 1996

Caine ED: Gilles de la Tourette's syndrome: a review of clinical and research studies and consideration of future directions for investigation. Arch Neurol 42:393–397, 1985

Caine ED, Polinsky RJ, Ebert MH, et al: Trial of clomipramine and desipramine for Gilles de la Tourette syndrome. Ann Neurol 5:305–306, 1979

Carlsson M, Svensson K, Erikson E, et al: Rat brain serotonin: biochemical and functional evidence for a sex difference. J Neural Transm 63:297–313, 1985

Castellanos FX, Ritchie FG, Marsh WL, Rapoport JL. DSM-IV stereotypic movement disorder: persistence of stereotypies of infancy in intellectually normal adolescents and adults. J Clin Psychiatry 57:116–122, 1996

Christenson GA, Mackenzie TB, Mitchell JE. Characteristics of 60 adult chronic hair pullers. Am J Psychiatry 148:365–370, 1991a

Christenson GA, Popkin MK, Mackenzie TB, et al: Lithium treatment of chronic hair pulling. J Clin Psychiatry 52:116–120, 1991b

Christenson GA, Mackenzie TB, Mitchell JE, et al: A placebo-controlled, double-blind crossover study of fluoxetine in trichotillomania. Am J Psychiatry 148:1566–1571, 1991c

Christenson GA, Mackenzie TB, Reeve EA: Familial trichotillomania (letter). Am J Psychiatry 149:283, 1992

Christenson GA, Raymond NC, Faris PL, et al: Pain thresholds are not elevated in trichotillomania. Biol Psychiatry 36:347–349, 1994

Christenson GA, Crow JC, Mackenzie TB: A placebo controlled double-blind study of naltrexone for trichotillomania. Presented at the Annual Meeting of the American Psychiatric Association, Miami, Florida, May 1995

Christenson GA, Crow SJ, Mitchell JE, et al: Fluvoxamine in the treatment of trichotillomania: an 8-week, open-label study. CNS Spectrums 3:64–71, 1998

Cohen DJ, Detlor J, Young G, et al: Clonidine ameliorates Gilles de la Tourette syndrome. Arch Gen Psychiatry 37:1350–1357, 1980

Cohen LJ, Stein DJ, Simeon D, et al: Clinical profile, comorbidity, and treatment history in 123 hairpullers: a survey study. J Clin Psychiatry 36:319–326, 1995

Cooper SJ, Dourish CT (eds): Neurobiology of Stereotyped Behavior. New York, Oxford University Press, 1990

Cronin GM, Wiepkema PR, Van Ree JM: Endorphins implicated in stereotypies of tethered sows. Experientia 42:198–199, 1986

De Waal F: Good Natured: The Origins of Right and Wrong in Humans and Other Animals. Cambridge, MA, Harvard University Press, 1996

DeSimoni MG, Dal-Toso G, Fodritto F, et al: Modulation of striatal dopamine metabolism by the activity of dorsal raphe serotonergic afferences. Brain Res 411:81–88, 1987

Dillon JE: Self-injurious behavior associated with clonidine withdrawal in a child with Tourette's disorder. J Child Neurol 5:308–310, 1990

Dodman NH, Shuster L, White SD, et al: Use of narcotic agonists to modify stereotypic self-licking, self-chewing, and scratching behavior in dogs. J Am Vet Med Assoc 193:815–819, 1988

Dodman N, Moon A, Stein DJ: Animal models of obsessive-compulsive disorder, in Obsessive-Compulsive Disorders: Etiology, Diagnosis, Treatment. Edited by Hollander E, Stein DJ, New York, Marcel Decker, 1997, pp 99–144

Eapen V, Trimble MR, Robertson MM: The use of fluoxetine in Gilles de la Tourette syndrome and obsessive compulsive behaviors: preliminary clinical experience. Prog Neuropsychopharm Biol Psychiatry 20:737–743, 1996

Favazza AR: Bodies Under Siege. Baltimore, MD, The Johns Hopkins University Press, 1987

Friedman EH: Bradycardia and somnolence after adding fluoxetine to pimozide regimen. Can J Psychiatry 39:634, 1994

Goodman WK, McDougle CJ, Price LH, et al: Beyond the serotonin hypothesis: a role for dopamine in some forms of obsessive compulsive disorder? J Clin Psychiatry 51(suppl):36–43, 1990

Grindlinger HM, Ramsay E: Compulsive feather picking in birds. Arch Gen Psychiatry 48:857, 1991

Gupta MA, Gupta AK: Fluoxetine is an effective treatment for neurotic excoriations: case report. Cutis 51:386–387, 1993

Gupta MA, Gupta AK, Haberman HF: Neurotic excoriations: a review and some new perspectives. Compr Psychiatry 27:381–386, 1986

Haber SN, Kowall NW, Von Sattell, et al: Gilles de la Tourette's syndrome: a postmortem neuropathological and immunohistochemical study. J Neurol Sci 76:225–241, 1986

Hadley NH: Fingernail Biting: Theory, Research and Treatment. New York, Spectrum Publications, 1984

Hallopeau M: Alopecia par grottage (trichomania ou trichotillomania). Annales de Dermatologie et Venerologie 10:440–441, 1889

Hansen DJ, Tishelman AC, Hawkins RP, et al: Habits with potential as disorders: prevalence, severity, and other characteristics among college students. Behavior Modification 14:66–80, 1990

Hansen-Grant S, Silk KR, Guthrie S: Fluoxetine–pimozide interaction. Am J Psychiatry 150:1751–1752, 1994

Hartmann L: Cats as possible obsessive-compulsive disorder and medication models (letter). Am J Psychiatry 152:1236, 1995

Hawkridge S, Stein DJ, Bouwer C: Combining neuroleptics with serotonin specific reuptake inhibitors in Tourette's syndrome. J Am Acad Child Adolesc Psychiatry 35:703–704, 1996

Herman BH: A possible role of proopiomelanocortin peptides in self-injurious behavior. Prog Neuropsychopharmacol Biol Psychiatry 14S:109–139, 1990

Hollander E, Cohen L, Richards M, et al: A pilot study of the neuropsychology of obsessive-compulsive disorder and Parkinson's disease: basal ganglia disorders. J Neuropsychiatry Clin Neurosci 5:104–107, 1993

Hollander E, Stein DJ, DeCaria CM, et al: Serotonergic sensitivity in borderline personality disorder: preliminary findings. Am J Psychiatry 151:277–280, 1994

Horrigan JP, Barnhill LJ: Paroxetine-pimozide interaction. J Am Acad Child Adolesc Psychiatry 33:1060–1061, 1994

Hyde TM, Weinberger DR: Tourette's syndrome: a model neuropsychiatric disorder. JAMA 273:498–501, 1995

Hyde TM, Stacey ME, Coppola R, et al: Cerebral morphometric abnormalities in Tourette's syndrome: a quantitative MRI study of monozygotic twins. Neurology 1176–1182, 1995

Insel TR: Toward a neuroanatomy of obsessive-compulsive disorder. Arch Gen Psychiatry 49:739–744, 1992

Joubert CE: Relationship of self-esteem, manifest anxiety, and obsessive-compulsiveness to personal habits. Psychol Rep 73:579–583, 1993

Kalivas J, Kalivas L, Gilman D, et al: Sertraline in the treatment of neurotic excoriations and related disorders. Arch Dermatol 132:589–590, 1996

Katz RJ, Landau P, DeVeaugh-Geiss J, et al: Pharmacological responsiveness of dermatitis secondary to compulsive washing. Psych Res 34:223–226, 1990

Keuthen NJ, Savage CR, O'Sullivan RL, et al: Neuropsychological functioning in trichotillomania. Biol Psychiatry 39:747–749, 1996

Keuthen NJ, O'Sullivan RL, Goodchild P, et al: Retrospective review of treatment outcome in 63 patients with trichotillomania. Am J Psychiatry 155:560–561, 1998

Koran LM, Ringold A, Hewlett W. Fluoxetine for trichotillomania: an open clinical trial. Psychopharmacol Bull 28:145–149, 1992

Kurlan R, Como PG, Deeley C, et al: A pilot controlled study of fluoxetine for obsessive-compulsive symptoms in children with Tourette's syndrome. Clin Neuropharmacol 16:167–172, 1993

Leckman JF: What genes confer vulnerability to Gilles de la Tourette's syndrome? Psychiatr Ann 27:293–296, 1997

Leckman JF, Ort S, Caruso KA, et al: Rebound phenomena in Tourette's syndrome after abrupt withdrawal of clonidine: behavioral, cardiovascular, and neurochemical effects. Arch Gen Psychiatry 43:1168–1176, 1986

Leckman JF, Riddle MA, Berrettini WH, et al: Elevated CSF dynorphin A[1–8] in Tourette's syndrome. Life Sci 43:2015–2023, 1988

Leckman JF, Walker DE, Cohen DJ: Premonitory urges in Tourette's syndrome. Am J Psychiatry 150:98–102, 1993

Leckman JF, Goodman WK, Anderson GM, et al: Cerebrospinal fluid biogenic amines in obsessive-compulsive disorder, Tourette's syndrome, and healthy controls. Neuropsychopharmacology 12:73–86, 1995

Lenane MC, Swedo SE, Rapoport JL, et al: Rates of obsessive compulsive disorder in first degree relatives of patients with trichotillomania: a research note. J Child Psychol Psychiatry 33:925–933, 1992

Leonard HL, Swedo SE, Rapoport JL, et al: Treatment of obsessive-compulsive disorder with clomipramine and desipramine in children and adolescents: a double-blind crossover comparison. Arch Gen Psychiatry 46:1088–1092, 1989

Leonard HL, Lenane MC, Swedo SE, et al: A double-blind comparison of clomipramine and desipramine treatment of severe onychophagia (nail biting). Arch Gen Psychiatry 48:821–827, 1991

MacLean PD: Effects of lesions of globus pallidus on species-typical display behavior of squirrel monkeys. Brain Res 149:175–196, 1978

Malison RT, McDougle CJ, van Dyck CH, et al: [123I]B-CIT SPECT imaging of striatal dopamine transporter binding in Tourette's disorder. Am J Psychiatry 152:1359–1361, 1995

Martin A, Scahill L, Vitulani L, King A: Stimulant use and trichotillomania. J Am Acad Child Adolesc Psychiatry 37:349–350, 1998

Martin LJ, Spicer DM, Lewis MH, et al: Social deprivation of infant monkeys alters the hemoarchitecture of the brain, I: subcortical regions. J Neurosci 11:3344–3358, 1991

McConville BJ, Norman AB, Fogelson MH, et al: Sequential use of opioid antagonists and agonists in Tourette's syndrome. Lancet 343:601, 1994

McDougle CJ, Goodman WK, Leckman JF, et al: Haloperidol addition in fluvoxamine-refractory obsessive-compulsive disorder: a double-blind placebo-controlled study in patients with and without tics. Arch Gen Psychiatry 51:302–308, 1994

Mehregan AH: Trichotillomania: a clinicopathological study. Arch Dermatol 102:129–133, 1970

Muller SA: Trichotillomania. Dermatol Clin 5:595–601, 1987

Neziroglu F, Anemone R, Yaryura-Tobias JA: Onset of obsessive-compulsive disorder in pregnancy. Am J Psychiatry 149:947–950, 1992

Niehaus DJ, Emsley RA, Brink PA, et al: Stereotypies: prevalence and association with compulsive and impulsive symptoms in college students. Psychopathology 33:31–35, 2000

Ninan PT, Rothbaum BO, Stipetic M, et al: CSF 5HIAA as a predictor of treatment response in trichotillomania. Psychopharmacol Bull 28:451–455, 1992

O'Sullivan RL, Rauch SL, Breiter HC, et al: Reduced basal ganglia volumes in trichotillomania measured by morphometric magnetic resonance imaging. Biol Psychiatry 42:39–45,1997

O'Sullivan RL, Keuthen NJ, Rodriguez D, et al: Venlafaxine treatment of trichotillomania: an open case series of ten cases. CNS Spectrums 3:56–63, 1998

Pauls DL, Towbin KE, Leckman JF, et al: Gilles de la Tourette's syndrome and obsessive-compulsive disorder: evidence supporting a genetic relationship. Arch Gen Psychiatry 43:1180–1182, 1986

Peterson B, Leckman JF, Scahill L, et al: Hypothesis: steroid hormones and CNS sexual dimorphisms modulate symptom expression in Tourette's syndrome. Psychoneuroendocrinology 17:553–563, 1993a

Peterson B, Riddle MA, Cohen DJ, et al: Reduced basal ganglia volumes in Tourette's syndrome using three-dimensional reconstruction techniques from magnetic resonance images. Neurology 43:941–949, 1993b

Peterson B, Leckman JF, Scahill L, et al: Steroid hormones and Tourette's syndrome: early experience with antiandrogen therapy. J Clin Psychopharm 14:131–135, 1994

Phillips KA, Taub SL: Skin picking as a symptom of body dysmorphic disorder. Psychopharmacol Bull 31:279–288, 1995

Pitman RK, Green RC, Jenike MA, et al: Clinical comparison of Tourette's disorder and obsessive-compulsive disorder. Am J Psychiatry 144:1166–1171, 1987

Pollard CA, Ibe IO, Krojanker DN, et al: Clomipramine treatment of trichotillomania: a follow-up report on four cases. J Clin Psychiatry 52:128–130, 1991

Potenza MN, Waslink S, Epperson CN, et al: Olanzapine augmentation of fluoxetine in the treatment of trichotillomania. Am J Psychiatry 155:1299–1300, 1998

Primeau F, Fontaine R: Obsessive disorder with self-mutilation: a subgroup responsive to pharmacotherapy. Can J Psychiatry 32:699–700, 1987

Rapoport JL, Ryland DH, Kriete M: Drug treatment of canine acral lick: an animal model of obsessive-compulsive disorder. Arch Gen Psychiatry 48:517–521, 1992

Rasmusson AM, Anderson GM, Lynch KA, et al: A preliminary study of tryptophan depletion on tics, obsessive-compulsive symptoms, and mood in Tourette's syndrome. Biol Psychiatry 41:117–121, 1997

Rettew DC, Cheslow DL, Rapoport JL, et al: Neuropsychological test performance in trichotillomania: a further link with obsessive-compulsive disorder. J Anxiety Disord 5:225–235, 1991

Robertson MM: The Gilles de la Tourette Syndrome: the current status. Br J Psychiatry 154:147–169, 1989

Robertson MM, Trimble MR, Lees A: Self-injurious behavior and the Gilles de la Tourette syndrome: a clinical study and review of the literature. Psychol Med 19:611–625, 1989

Robertson M, Doran M, Trimble M, et al: The treatment of Gilles de la Tourette syndrome by limbic leucotomy. J Neurol Neurosurg Psychiatry 53:691–694, 1990

Rodrigo-Escalona-P, Adair JC, Roberts BB, et al: Obsessive-compulsive disorder following bilateral global pallidus infarction. Biol Psychiatry 42:410–412, 1997

Seedat S, Stein DJ: Psychosocial and economic implications of trichotillomania: a pilot study in a South African sample. CNS Spectrums 3:40–43, 1998

Shapiro AK, Shapiro E: Tourette syndrome: clinical aspects, treatment, and etiology. Semin Neurol 2:373–385, 1982

Sheika SH, Wagner KD, Wagner RF Jr.: Fluoxetine treatment of trichotillomania and depression in a prepubertal child. Cutis 51:50–52, 1993

Simeon D, Cohen LJ, Stein DJ, et al: Comorbid self-injurious behaviors in 71 female hair-pullers: a survey study. J Nerv Ment Dis 185:117–119, 1997a

Simeon D, Stein DJ, Gross S, et al: A double-blind trial of fluoxetine in pathologic skin picking. J Clin Psychiatry 58:341–347, 1997b

Singer HS, Hahn IH, Moran TH: Abnormal dopamine uptake sites in postmortem striatum from patients with Tourette's syndrome. Ann Neurol 30:558–562, 1991

Singer HS, Reiss AL, Brown JE, et al: Volumetric MRI changes in basal ganglia of children with Tourette's syndrome. Neurology 43:950–956, 1993

Soriano JL, O'Sullivan RL, Baer L, et al: Trichotillomania and self-esteem: a survey of 62 female hair pullers. J Clin Psychiatry 57:77–82, 1996

Stanley MA, Bowers TC, Swann AC, et al: Treatment of trichotillomania with fluoxetine (letter). J Clin Psychiatry 52:282, 1991

Stein DJ, Hollander E: Dermatology and conditions related to obsessive-compulsive disorder. J Am Acad Dermatol 26:237–242, 1992a

Stein DJ, Hollander E: Low-dose pimozide augmentation of serotonin reuptake blockers in the treatment of trichotillomania. J Clin Psychiatry 53:123–126, 1992b

Stein DJ, Hollander E: The spectrum of obsessive-compulsive related disorders, in Obsessive-Compulsive Related Disorders. Edited by Hollander E. Washington, DC, American Psychiatric Press, 1993, pp 241–271

Stein DJ, Simeon D: Pharmacotherapy of stereotypic movement disorders. Psychiatr Ann 28:327–334, 1998

Stein DJ, Hutt CS, Spitz JL, et al: Compulsive picking and obsessive-compulsive disorder. Psychosomatics 34:177-181, 1993

Stein DJ, Hollander E, Simeon D, et al: Neurological soft signs in female patients with trichotillomania. J Neuropsychiatry Clin Neurosci 6:184–187, 1994

Stein DJ, Hollander E, Cohen L, et al: Serotonergic responsivity in trichotillomania: neuroendocrine effects of M-chlorophenylpiperazine. Biol Psychiatry 37:414–416, 1995

Stein DJ, Hollander E, Simeon D, et al: Behavioral responses to M-chlorophenylpiperazine and clonidine in trichotillomania. J Serotonin Res 4:11–15, 1997a

Stein DJ, Wessels C, Carr J, et al: Hair-pulling in a patient with Sydenham's chorea. Am J Psychiatry 154:1320, 1997b

Stein DJ, Coetzer R, Lee M, et al: Magnetic resonance brain imaging in women with obsessive-compulsive disorder and trichotillomania. Psychiatry Res 74:177–182, 1997c

Stein DJ, Bouwer C, Hawkridge S, et al: Risperidone augmentation of serotonin reuptake inhibitors in obsessive-compulsive and related disorders. J Clin Psychiatry 58:119–122, 1997d

Stein DJ, Bouwer C, Niehaus D: Stereotypic movement disorder. J Clin Psychiatry 58:177–178, 1997e

Stein DJ, Bouwer C, Maud CM: Use of the selective serotonin reuptake inhibitor citalopram in the treatment of trichotillomania. Eur Arch Psychiatry Clin Neurosci 247:234–236, 1997f

Stein DJ, van Heerden B, Wessels C, et al: Functional imaging and medication in hairpulling. Presented at the Annual Meeting of the American Psychiatric Association, San Diego, CA, June 1998a

Stein DJ, O' Sullivan R, Hollander E: Neurobiology of trichotillomania, in Tricho-tillomania: Current Concepts. Edited by Stein DJ, Christenson GA, Hollander E. Washington, DC, American Psychiatric Press, 1998b, pp 43–61

Stein DJ, Niehaus DJH, Seedat S, et al: Phenomenology of stereotypic movement disorder. Psychiatr Ann 28:307–312, 1998c

Stout RJ: Fluoxetine for the treatment of compulsive facial picking (letter). Am J Psychiatry 147:370, 1990

Streichenwein SM, Thornby JI: A long-term, double-blind, placebo-controlled crossover trial of the efficacy of fluoxetine for trichotillomania. Am J Psychiatry 148:1566–1571, 1995

Swanepoel N, Lee E, Stein DJ: Psychogenic alopecia in a cat: response to clomi-pramine. South Africa Journal of Veterinary Medicine 69:22, 1998

Swedo SE, Schapiro MB, Grady CL, et al: Cerebral glucose metabolism in child-hood-onset obsessive-compulsive disorder. Arch Gen Psychiatry 46:518–523, 1989a

Swedo SE, Leonard HL, Rapoport JL, et al: A double-blind comparison of clomi-pramine and desipramine in the treatment of trichotillomania (hair pulling). N Engl J Med 321:497–501, 1989b

Swedo SE, Rapoport JL, Leonard HL, et al: Regional cerebral glucose metabolism of women with trichotillomania. Arch Gen Psychiatry 48:828–833, 1991

Swedo SE, Leonard HL, Lenane MC, et al: Trichotillomania: a profile of the disor-der from infancy through adulthood. Int Pediatr 7:144–150, 1992

Swedo SE, Lenane MC, Leonard HL: Long-term treatment of trichotillomania. N Engl J Med 329:141–142, 1993

Swedo SE, Leonard HL, Mittleman BB, et al: Identification of children with pediat-ric autoimmune neuropsychiatric disorders associated with streptococcal in-fections by a marker associated with rheumatic fever. Am J Psychiatry 154:110–112, 1997

Thoren P, Asberg M, Bertilsson L, et al: Clomipramine treatment of obsessive-compulsive disorder, II: biochemical aspects. Arch Gen Psychiatry 37:1289–1294, 1980

Traber J, Spencer DG, Glaser T, et al: Actions of psychoactive drugs on ACTH- and novelty-induced behavior in the rat. Ann N Y Acad Sci 525:270–280, 1988

van Ameringen M, Mancini C: Treatment of trichotillomania with haloperidol. Anxiety Disorders Association of America Annual Meeting. Orlando, FL, 1996

Willemse T, Muddle M, Josephy M, et al: The effect of haldol and naloxone on ex-cessive grooming behavior of cats. Eur Neuropsychopharmacol 4:39–45, 1994

Winchel RM, Jones JS, Stanley B, et al: Clinical characteristics of trichotillomania and its response to fluoxetine. J Clin Psychiatry 53:304–308, 1992

Wolf SS, Jones DW, Knable MB, et al: Tourette syndrome: prediction of phenotypic variation in monozygotic twins by caudate nucleus D2 receptor binding. Sci-ence 273:1225–1227, 1996

Zohar J, Insel TR: Obsessive-compulsive disorder: psychobiological approaches to diagnosis, treatment, and pathophysiology. Biol Psychiatry 22:667–687, 1987

# CHAPTER 5

# Psychotherapies for Compulsive Self-Injurious Behaviors

Bonnie Aronowitz, Ph.D.

*T*he range of compulsive self-injurious behaviors (SIBs) is described in Chapter 1. There is a notable absence of controlled empirical treatment studies in the field of compulsive SIB; thus, existing treatments in the literature consisting largely of case studies, case series, and behavioral techniques are presented in this chapter. Trichotillomania, or compulsive hair pulling, is the most widely addressed in the literature and will thus be the main focus, followed by a brief review of the treatment of skin picking and onychophagia.

## Trichotillomania

### Psychoanalytic Perspectives

The earliest authors first described patients with trichotillomania as otherwise "sane" (Hallopeau 1889). However, later psychoanalytic literature, composed of clinical observational data and single case studies, has conceptualized patients with the disorder as having a profound disturbance (Mannino and Delgado 1969) and the actual hair pulling behavior as highly treatment refractory (Greenberg and Sarner 1965). Hair pulling has been viewed as having specific or multiple (Krishnan et al. 1985) unconscious symbolic meanings, such as beauty, bisexuality, physical prowess, and virility. Trichotillomania has also been viewed as a pathologic release mechanism (Mannino and Delgado 1969) for either erotic (Masserman 1955; Zaidens 1951) or aggressive impulses (Fenichel 1945; Irwin 1953) or as the result of pathologic psychosexual development (Greenberg 1969). Krishnan et al. (1985) conceptualized sexual conflicts as being displaced onto the hair and viewed haircutting or plucking as being symbolic of castration. The origin of trichotillomania has been postulated as resulting from specific familial constellations such as disordered mother–child relationships (Aleksandrowicz and Mares 1978; Singh and Maguire 1989); having an ambivalent, double-binding, aggressive mother and a passive, rejecting father; or being subjected to traumatic experiences such as incest (Oguchi and Miura 1977). Object relations theorists (Buxbaum 1960) identified hair pulling as an attempt to work through difficulties with object relationships using the hair as a transitional object.

Psychoanalytic case reports of patients with trichotillomania have reported a positive response to psychoanalytically oriented psychotherapy (Greenberg and Sarner 1965; Langford 1955; Monroe and Abse 1963). However, the general consensus in the current literature is that treatment should be directed at the hair pulling symptom itself rather than by diffusely concentrating on psychodynamic themes.

## Trichotillomania Treatment Studies

There are nearly as many treatment modalities in the literature on trichotillomania as there are actual articles on the topic. Most of these studies claim efficacy and are case presentations instead of controlled studies. The measurement of improvement in published treatment outcome studies has varied widely, with many uncontrolled case studies relying solely on impressionistic indices of improvement that are devoid of adequate empirical validation. Treatment includes the phases of assessment, accurate diagnosis, psychoeducation, self-monitoring, self-management, and self-maintenance. Current treatment options include various pharmacologic treatments (described in Chapter 4), behavioral techniques, and hypnosis.

## Behavioral Treatments

Behavioral techniques cited in the literature typically are characterized by highly motivated, capable, compliant patients actively seeking treatment who can practice homeworks and perform self-administered techniques (Risch and Ferguson 1981). Thus, behavioral treatment studies should be interpreted in light of the fact that samples may constitute a selection bias in favor of higher-functioning individuals and therefore claims of efficacy may not be generalizable to the trichotillomania population at large. Moreover, the necessary and sufficient ingredients of treatments, particularly when used in combination, have yet to be ascertained.

The following is a classification of the behavioral techniques used to treat trichotillomania in adults, children, and the developmentally disabled. A brief methodologic review of these behavioral techniques follows their description (Aronowitz and Josephson 1996; Keuthen et al. 1999). The isolation of techniques is somewhat artificial for the sake of illustrative purposes; in practice, most techniques are used in combination or in treatment packages.

## Self-Monitoring

Self-monitoring (Bayer 1972) in trichotillomania treatment aims to provide baseline and continuous data about the patient's hair pulling behavior and urges through increases in self-awareness of the behavior. Recording hair pulling to increase self-awareness can be extended to a technique called *awareness training*, in which the patient records instances of hair pulling in addition to activities and emotions during both hair pulling urges and actual hair pulling. The intent is to interrupt the seemingly automatic chain of trichotillomanic behavior. Ottens (1982) stressed heightening patients' awareness of the overt and covert behaviors that are precursors to pulling in addition to the hair pulling behavior itself. Awareness training helps patients identify their hair pulling patterns and initiates discussion of compliance and motivation issues. Because self-monitoring as a sole treatment method has largely been conducted in case studies, it cannot be reliably assessed. In their analysis of 75 chronic hair pullers, in which they identified relevant cues for trichotillomanic episodes, Christenson et al. (1993) found the components of negative affective states, sedentary activities, and contemplative attitudes to be core features of such episodes. Such studies are important in the further elucidation of the triggers of trichotillomania.

Most investigators have combined self-monitoring with other behavioral treatment components such as mild aversion treatment (Stevens 1984) and mild aversive self-control, such as saving hairs for the therapist (Bayer 1972), and found such combinations to increase responsibility for pulling and to generally enhance treatment effects (Friman et al. 1984). No published group study or well-controlled, single-subject experimental design study has investigated the independent efficacy of self-monitoring. Wolfsohn and Barling (1978) and Stabler and Warren (1974) required patients to both self-monitor and to collect all hairs pulled. Bayer (1972) found that the degree of the therapist's involvement in the collection of hairs pulled determined the degree of efficacy of this technique. Thus, greater the involvement of the therapist, such as in viewing pulled hairs brought to the session, resulted in better outcome than simple patient monitoring of hairs pulled. This is intuitively appealing because accountability has been demonstrated to enhance treatment effects for target behaviors in most behavioral treatments.

## Habit Reversal

The most thoroughly evaluated behavioral therapy for trichotillomania is habit reversal (Azrin and Nunn 1973). Habit reversal and its variants (Rosenbaum and Ayllon 1981) have been termed the most successful self-management techniques for trichotillomania by some authors (Winchel 1992). In this technique, the patient receives habit awareness training and practices competing motor responses incompatible with the target hair pulling behavior in order to inhibit pulling. Habit reversal aims to interrupt the target behavior, prevent additional hair pulling, and develop an opposing behavior.

Azrin et al. (1980b) randomly assigned 34 subjects to either a habit reversal ($n=19$) or negative practice group ($n=15$). Thirty-two subjects recorded each hair pulling occurrence; two recorded duration instead of number because the habit was continuous rather than episodic. Subjects in the habit reversal group were taught a competing response of 3-minute fist clenching at the onset of pulling urges. Subjects in the negative practice group were instructed to stand in front of a mirror hourly and act out hair pulling motions for 30 seconds without actual pulling. Habit reversal reduced hair pulling in excess of 90%, whereas negative practice reduced pulling by only 50%.

The Azrin et al. (1980b) study is the only published randomized group study of behavior therapy in trichotillomania. Other case studies and single-subject experimental designs have supported the findings of this study, but additional controlled studies are required for its replication. Rosenbaum and Ayllon (1981) supported Azrin et al.'s findings in a four-subject study. Other authors, by component analyses, have attempted to isolate necessary and sufficient conditions for the treatment success of Azrin et al.'s habit reversal paradigm for habit disorders, but they did not specifically focus on trichotillomania (Horne and Wilkinson 1980; Ladouceur 1979; Miltenberger and Fuqua 1985; Miltenberger et al. 1985; Ollendick 1981).

It is generally agreed that habit reversal may essentially be considered a treatment package consisting of up to 13 components (Tarnowski et al. 1987). It comprises training in self-monitoring, competing responses, and relaxation as well as recruitment of social support and habit inconvenience review or the delineation of the negative effects of the habit on one's lifestyle (Finney et al. 1983). Habit interruption, practice of competing responses, and prevention training (Tarnowski et al. 1987) were additional components.

## Classical Conditioning

**Reinforcement.** Reinforcement has been used in a number of treatment-outcome studies of trichotillomania and is usually added to other behavioral strategies. Reinforcement may take the form of attention, hugs, praise (Saper 1971), and token economies (Wolfsohn and Barling 1978), in which subjects receive actual rewards for refraining from hair pulling. Case studies have found reinforcement to be effective, particularly in children. However, because randomized group studies were not conducted with reinforcement as the primary or sole treatment, its efficacy cannot be determined.

**In Vivo Versus Imaginal Exposure and Response Prevention.** With in vivo exposure, the patient is placed in a stressful situation that typically results in a hair pulling response; this response is then prevented. In imaginal exposure, the patient is told to imagine a stressful situation that commonly leads to hair pulling; this is then followed by hair pulling prevention. Another method of hair pulling response prevention involves cutting hair very close to the scalp (Massong et al. 1980).

## Operant Conditioning

**Punishment/Aversive Techniques.** Punishment and other aversive behavioral techniques have been reported to result in significant reduction of hair pulling. Punishment has included self-imposed consequences such as the self-administration of a rubber band snap (Mastellone 1974), application of aversive eye drops for eyelash pulling (Epstein and Peterson 1973), and rigorous exercise with the onset of hair pulling urges (MacNeil and Thomas 1976). Response cost, considered a relatively milder aversive treatment technique, is the self-denial of privileges contingent on hair pulling episodes (Bayer 1972; Cordle and Long 1980; Horne 1977; MacNeil and Thomas 1976).

Punishment has also included consequences imposed by others such as ammonia inhalation; verbal reprimands; application of aversive taste substances to the thumb if thumb sucking is a covarying habit disorder; electrical aversion therapy and facial screening; or placing a soft cloth over the face. Multiple case studies and single-subject designs have reported on the use of punishment as a behavioral treatment for trichotillomania, but because controlled studies are lacking, definitive statements cannot be made about the efficacy of punishment.

Behavioral contracting (Stabler and Warren 1974) involves verbal or written contracts between patients and their therapists in which patients promise to refrain from hair pulling according to a mutually agreed upon plan. Contracting may also provide a powerful form of social reinforcement and approval.

Pharmacologic pain sensitization has recently been employed in the treatment of trichotillomania (Ristvedt and Christenson 1996). The rationale for the procedure is that patients experience no discomfort during trichotillomanic episodes, which thus enables them to engage in hair pulling outside of consciousness. The authors used a topical cream to enhance pain sensitivity in one case study. The increased pain sensitization, in conjunction with a habit reversal technique, resulted in markedly decreased hair pulling.

**Overcorrection.**   Overcorrection has been termed a punishment procedure that involves practicing overly correct versions of a behavior contingent upon a target response (e.g., properly brushing or combing the area of hair pulled, either on a daily basis or after each episode of pulling) (Foxx and Bechtel 1982). Unfortunately, this procedure can cause hair loss (Steck 1979) and may be perceived by patients as extremely stressful. Overcorrection may be used as a positive practice to train hair pullers to engage in appropriate handling of their hair (Vitulano et al. 1992), or as a punishment procedure used to decrease hair pulling in developmentally delayed individuals.

Barrett and Shapiro (1980) reported the use of overcorrection for the treatment of hair pulling in a 7½-year-old severely mentally retarded girl. After observing no reduction in hair pulling as a result of verbal warnings, the girl was instructed to brush her hair appropriately for 2-minute periods following each hair pulling instance. A near zero rate of hair pulling was achieved with the use of this technique.

Other multicomponent treatment packages may include behavioral techniques used in conjunction with various other therapies, including reinforcement and response cost followed by self-instruction (Wolfsohn and Barling 1978); cognitive desensitization (Meichenbaum 1972) with self-monitoring; relaxation; goal setting (Bornstein and Rychtarik (1978); attention-reflection and punishment (Altman et al. 1982); habit reversal; stimulus control; cognitive techniques; and role-play (Rothbaum 1992).

**Covert Desensitization.**   An additional form of operant conditioning with a more covert punishing agent is termed *covert desensitization*. Patients using covert desensitization punish their urges and actual hair pulling behaviors either in their imaginations or covertly—for example, by conjuring the image of a greatly distressing or anxiety-provoking event with the urge to hair pull (Cautela 1967). Examples of such images include visualizing part of their scalps being yanked out with each hair pull and the resulting blood, infection, nausea, and vomiting. Case studies that employed this technique alone or in combination with other techniques have reported therapeutic efficacy for trichotillomania, which has been maintained at follow-up (Levine 1976). Levine (1976) first reported the use of covert desensitization to treat trichotillomania in his case study of an adult hair puller previously treated for 5 years in unsuccessful analytic treatment. With covert desensitization, hair pulling dropped to zero rates that were maintained at follow-up. Because few studies have reported on covert desensitization as a behavioral treatment for trichotillomania and it has not been used in controlled studies, its efficacy is not possible to determine.

## Cognitive and Behavioral Treatments

Cognitive-behavioral therapy, in addition to exerting therapeutic efforts on the hair pulling behavior itself, addresses the cognitive component of such behavior as pivotal for producing change. Cognitive treatments include challenging cognitive-mediating influences on patients' trichotillomania, such as attributions, self-statements, anxiety, and anger-inducing cognitions that often precipitate hair pulling episodes (Ottens 1981). In addition to treatment by competing response methodology, Ottens teaches patients cognitive coping skills or positive self-statements such as appropriate self-instruction, covert assertion, rational disputation of irrational thoughts, and anticipatory strategies. These cognitive coping skills counteract the automatic negative thoughts patients have before and during hair pulling episodes.

Cognitive-behavioral treatments have also been used in combination with other techniques. McLaughlin and Nay (1975) used relaxation, self-monitoring, and cognitive-behavioral self-statements. Taylor (1963) used self-administered negative reinforcement and cognitive self-statements such as thought-stopping (e.g., interruption of the thought by an appropriate self-statement such as "stop now!").

Rational-emotive therapy is a type of cognitive-behavioral treatment that aims to identify maladaptive thought patterns hypothesized as causing the anxiety states that lead to hair pulling. Bernard et al. (1983) found this technique to be of modest benefit in the treatment of trichotillomania; when self-instructional training was added, hair pulling was rapidly eliminated. These benefits were maintained at 5- and 21-week follow-up evaluations.

## Relaxation and Hypnosis

No controlled studies have been made of hypnotherapy in the treatment of trichotillomania, but case reports claim benefits from this technique

(Barabasz 1987; Gardner 1978; Horne 1977). Typically, the inducible patient is provided with posthypnotic suggestions about having control over hair pulling behavior. Other authors found only short-term benefits from hypnotherapy in some trichotillomania patients. Patients with partial benefits from either hypnosis or medication alone appear to fare better with a combination of both techniques (Winchel 1992).

De Luca and Holborn (1984) compared relaxation training and aforementioned habit reversal in the treatment of hair pulling. Relaxation consisted of the systematic tensing and relaxation of muscles (Wolpe 1973) twice weekly for several weeks. Relaxation was initially effective in hair pulling reduction but did not provide long-term benefit. In contrast, habit reversal had enduring effects in trichotillomania cessation.

### Behavior Therapy Versus Pharmacotherapy

A single treatment modality alone may not be enough to provide benefit to patients with refractory trichotillomania. In such cases, a combination of both behavioral and pharmacologic treatments may be indicated. Rothbaum and Ninan (1992), using a double-blind paradigm, randomized 14 patients with trichotillomania to 9-week trials of clomipramine (up to 250 mg/day), cognitive-behavioral treatment, or placebo. The cognitive-behavioral treatment consisted of habit reversal training and stimulus control to control hair pulling behavior, stress inoculation training for stress management, and relapse prevention to maintain gains. This group demonstrated significantly greater improvement both in trichotillomania symptom severity and functional impairment compared with the placebo group ($P<0.005$), which was maintained at 3-month follow-up. The clomipramine group had intermediate gains but tended to relapse when off medication, whereas the placebo group was unavailable for follow-up. Moreover, the combined treatment condition of pharmacotherapy plus behavior therapy is required to ascertain increased benefits of treatment combinations and to determine the relative contribution of each technique to the maintenance of treatment gains.

### Trichotillomania Treatment in Special Populations

#### Developmentally Disabled

Aversive techniques and punishment frequently have been used to treat trichotillomania in developmentally disabled (including autistic) individuals (Friman and Lucas 1994). Corte et al. (1971) used contingent electric shock therapy on a female adolescent with profound mental retardation.

Altman et al. (1978) used differential reinforcement of other behavior and response-contingent ammonia inhalation on a 4-year-old girl with severe retardation. Aforementioned overcorrection, the milder form of punishment used with developmentally delayed subjects (Barrett and Shapiro 1980; Matson et al. 1978), also has been found to significantly decrease hair pulling.

In a multiple baseline design, Barmann and Vitali (1982) used facial screening with three moderately to severely retarded, developmentally delayed child hair pullers. In this technique the patient's face and hair is briefly covered with a soft cloth bib when hair pulling occurs. The frequency of hair pulling was reduced in all three subjects by 86%, 66%, and 55%, respectively, from baseline conditions. Facial screening simultaneously produces response prevention, time out, and sensory extinction and is considered one of the least aversive punishments used for trichotillomania with a developmentally delayed population. Treatment combinations have included the use of facial screening. For example, Gross et al. (1982) used overcorrection with facial screening and differential reinforcement of other behavior on a 4-year-old with mild retardation.

### Children/Adolescents

Winchel (1992) advised that although implementation of behavioral approaches is particularly relevant to children, a conservative approach for medication in childhood trichotillomania should be followed. Most treatments for childhood trichotillomania have required implementation by parents or caregivers, such as reinforcement techniques requiring parents to provide daily attention, reflection, and periods of nonevaluative noncontingent play (Forehand and King (1974). Rosenbaum (1982) described a modified version of habit reversal for the treatment of recalcitrant childhood trichotillomania. Techniques of token economy combined with time out in a home-based treatment have also been used (Evans 1976).

## Skin Picking and Nail Biting

### Psychodynamically Oriented Treatment

Psychodynamic treatments or behavioral case reports of skin picking have yielded equivocal findings (Fruensgaard 1991a, 1991b; Koblenzer 1986; Seitz 1953; Welkowitz et al. 1989; Zaidens 1964). Psychotherapy has been used effectively for certain dermatoses (Koblenzer 1986), but it is an expensive and lengthy process subject to varied results because of patients' differing resistances to the exploration of underlying issues. Seitz (1953)

identified the main difficulties in psychodynamic treatment as the definition and diagnosis of neurotic excoriaton, patient selection, and relevant
follow-up evaluation. Fruensgaard (1991a; 1991b) conducted a multifacto-
rial investigation of psychodynamically oriented psychotherapy in 63 con-
secutive first-time referrals of neurotic excoriaton to a university hospital
dermatology department. Excoriation healed for 13 of the 63 patients at
1–5-year follow-up examination.

Honigl et al. (1997) believed that a disturbed relationship with one's
own body and with others is the etiology of neurotic excoriation. Deprivation and physical or sexual abuse were common in the histories of these
patients. Feelings of emptiness and unbearable psychic tension were identified as the immediate psychodynamic causes of the self-damaging act.
Psychotherapeutic strategies thought to be effective included learning to
express emotions in an enhanced manner, learning to care for one's own
body, and establishing confidential and stable relationships. Effective
therapeutic response to trauma survivors engaging in self-injury was
identified as particularly challenging. Appropriate clinical responses were
outlined by Connors (1996), including remaining present and open to
communication about disclosures of self-injury, helping patients intervene
in their own process of self-injury, and facilitating the resolution of underlying issues.

Psychoanalytic authors have contended that behaviors such as skin
biting or chewing have an erotic component (Obermayer 1955), but there
has been much disagreement about these interpretations (Scott and Scott
1997). Others refer to the oral-aggressive nature of nail biting (Koblenzer
1999). Various treatments for onychophagia have been reported in the literature including psychotherapy (Norton 1987), hypnosis (Bornstein et al.
1980), and relaxation training (Barrios 1977).

## Behavioral Interventions

The existing literature on behavioral techniques is limited to more severe
self-injury in developmentally disabled, mentally retarded, and autistic
samples. In these case studies, functional analysis of immediate antecedents and consequences to episodic self-injury produced inconclusive
results (O'Reilly 1996). Derby et al. (1996) described self-restraining and
self-injurious behaviors to be responses sometimes belonging to the same
functional response class—that is, maintained by identical contingency.
Thus, they hypothesized that a single treatment should prove effective for
both responses. They examined the effects of providing attention, the pre-
sumed reinforcer, both noncontingently and contingently upon either SIB

or self-restraint. Results were consistent with their hypothesis that both responses were maintained by attention and suggested that noncontingent reinforcement was a potentially effective treatment. Another case report suggested that self-restraint may be maintained using negative reinforcement in the form of escape from the aversive properties of SIBs such as pain. Fisher et al. (1996) examined the effects of blocking SIB on self-restraint. Consistent with the negative reinforcement hypothesis, blocking SIB resulted in near complete absence of SIB and moderate reductions in self-restraint.

Welkowitz et al. (1989) employed a multicomponent behavioral paradigm for neurotic scratching/neurotic excoriation in a case study. The treatment program consisted of self-monitoring/recording of scratching episodes, stimulus control procedures, and functional analysis. The goal was to separate a seemingly automatic behavior of scratching into its component elements and to promote instructional procedures for controlling these elements. This model assumed that excoriation is sometimes an automatic behavior that can be "unlearned."

Treatment of covert SIBs is complicated because of the difficulty in quantifying and applying differential consequences to covert responses. Grace et al. (1996) provided both tangible and social reinforcers contingent on the absence of tissue damage identified during physical examinations. This technique resulted in near 100% success in physical assessment checks maintained over 10-month follow-up.

Aronowitz (unpublished data, 1998) conducted a case series of 20 consecutively selected 20–50-year-old healthy female skin pickers presenting to clinical practice. Behavioral components included detailed self-monitoring, covering of mirrors followed by gradual exposure to mirrors, and response prevention of picking. In addition, the initial covering of hands with latex gloves was followed by gradual desensitization to uncovering. Cognitive techniques of response cost, imagery, and thought stopping were simultaneously employed. Structured relaxation and breathing training were added. Skin picking episodes were completely controlled in 15 patients with facial picking alone. The additional five patients with skin picking on other body parts had a 50% reduction in episode duration and severity of skin damage.

No systematic or controlled behavioral treatment studies have been conducted in onychophagia. Behavioral treatments that have resulted in short-term reduction of onychophagia include self-monitoring (Horan et al. 1974; Meade 1979), habit reversal (Azrin et al. 1980a), and negative practice (Azrin et al. 1980a; Smith 1978). Additional behavioral techniques include competing responses (Azrin et al. 1980a; DeLuca and Holborn

1984); overcorrection using artificial nails; and aversive techniques such as occlusive dressing or application of bitter substances, positive reinforcement (Davidson et al. 1980), covert sensitization (Daniels 1974; Paquin 1977), and behavioral contracting (Ross 1974).

There is an obvious need for enhanced understanding of the adaptive, ethologic, and psychodynamic significance and underlying psychobiology of compulsive habitual disorders and SIB. This may only be accomplished through systematic investigation from comparative studies. Behavioral treatments offer pragmatic, short-term treatments for compulsive and habit disorders. Component analysis of treatment packages and symptom severity is crucial in isolating effective treatment elements and their relative contributions to treatment outcome for these chronic and disabling disorders.

## Summary of Cognitive-Behavioral Treatments

Treatment modalities for compulsive SIB may vary widely in accordance with varying theoretical conceptualizations of the disorder. For example, psychoanalytic conceptualizations of self-injury may emphasize the origins of the disorder and the meanings of the behavior (e.g., underlying masochism). Psychologic bedrock is thought to be achieved when these repressed or unconscious etiologies are unearthed and have undergone psychoanalysis. Resultant motivational strength to tackle these dysfunctional masochistic behaviors is thus implicit in their understanding. In contrast, behavioral approaches place less emphasis on etiologic significance of SIBs and instead focus on the contingencies responsible for the onset, maintenance, and susceptibility to extinction of these behaviors.

Thus, theoretical constructions of self-injury may appear to exist in diametrical opposition. However, because of the incipient nature of moderate to severe self-injury and its associated functional impairment, many contemporary psychotherapists are actually eclectic in practice. Discerning clinicians should ascertain when they have reached the limits of their psychologic leverage with such patients, whether it be by the limits of interpretation or those of behavioral intervention. In patients with severe self-injury in which the automatic nature of the disorder is sufficiently inherent, pharmacotherapy may be a necessary prerequisite to either better regulate the intolerable affects underlying the self-injury or introduce a delay between impulse and motor action. More radically, successful phamacotherapy alone has been viewed as its own behavioral treatment in that the decrease or elimination of self-injury during a pharmacologic trial may involve covert learning of more adaptive responses. These adaptive responses are then retained, to varying degrees, in the patient's repertoire of competing behaviors against self-injury. Ideally, a concept of a significantly less- or non-self-injurious self is introduced; strong motivation to retain this self-concept may ensue.

Arguments abound regarding the ultimate therapeutic efficacy of the various interventions, especially in light of the fairly limited controlled treatment research in this area. For example, behavioral therapists contend that pharmacologic treatment would preclude patients' desensitization to all of the behavioral cues associated with the disorder. In this case, the self-injurious patient, if medicated, would be prevented from becoming habituated to intolerable affect contingencies responsible for the maintenance of the SIB. In contrast, phamacotherapists may argue that patients may be completely untreatable without adjunctive pharmacotherapy to minimally enable them to tolerate anxiety-provoking behavioral interventions.

Current treatment algorithms (Aronowitz and Hollander 1997) describe decision trees for good and poor responders to pharmacotherapy. For example, when behavioral treatment alone cannot be instituted because of low motivation, poor patient compliance, or severe symptoms, pharmacotherapy may be the sole recourse. Pharmacotherapy is typically recommended for a minimum of 1 year and behavioral treatment is added to this regimen as the patient begins to improve. Further behavioral treatment may then solidify the gains of pharmacotherapy, and the latter can consequently be phased out while behavioral intervention is retained for an additional year. Pharmacotherapy and behavioral intervention can thus be viewed as mutually facilitating. With continued poor response, augmentation of medication regimen with additional agents may be instituted, accompanied by a more aggressive behavioral regimen.

Regardless of the behavioral regimen instituted, the core ingredients culled from the treatment modalities described above are interpretation, self-monitoring, behavioral contracting, imagery, response prevention, and positive reinforcement. An example employing a combination of these techniques is illustrated in the following case.

### Case Example

The patient had engaged in 18 years of skin picking to the point of permanent scarring and infection; significant financial loss because of continuing dermatologic treatments and lost days of school and work; and extreme depression, agitation, and often dissociative episodes during and following the 2–15 hours frequently spent in front of the mirror. During severe self-mutilation episodes, the patient was housebound because of her disfigurement. Psychodynamic intervention included interpreting the patient's guilt about transcending her mother, who had been severely scarred for life by a disfiguring burn. Thus, the patient identified with her mother's shame and time-consuming cosmetic applications to camouflage scarring. In these ways, the patient enacted her conflicts about achievement—at times she successfully negotiated her life devoid of skin-picking episodes, and at other times she reverted to the identification with her mother and became housebound by self-inflicted wounds reminiscent of her mother's scarring.

The patient's gradual acceptance of such interpretations and consequent improved motivation resulted in self-monitoring of picking episodes and in behavioral contracting. However, with efforts to further achieve in her life, for example, new job interviews, test taking, and dating, the patient became so debilitated by the anxiety and dissociation of uncontrollable skin-picking episodes that she was unable to comply with behavioral assignments. Pharmacotherapy with fluoxetine was initiated, allowing her to successfully comply with graded exposure to the mirror and to implement response prevention. The patient was then better able to identify the contingencies responsible for the onset, maintenance, and cessation of the picking. Contingencies associated with initiation of the picking were the various opportunities of moving ahead with her career and romantic life. Contingencies associated with the maintenance of the picking included the initial damage done, time-consuming and costly but feeble attempts at repairing the damage, and ongoing anxiety associated with achievement. Cessation of the picking was associated with "irreparable damage" and fear of resultant suicide or institutionalization.

During pharmacotherapy, prevention of picking was accomplished first in the presence of the therapist for illustration of the technique and then in the presence of a trusted companion, who was instructed by the therapist in the methods of skin-picking coaching, such as how to get the patient away from the mirror. The goal was eventually to eliminate the patient's need of both the therapist and the companion. Positive reinforcement comprised engaging in activities that the patient enjoyed as a reward for not engaging in picking episodes. Negative reinforcement comprised the removal of agreed-upon activities of this nature following each picking episode.

When the patient was successfully able to prevent 95% of her skin-picking episodes, the companion was removed and the patient became self-reliant in the identification of cues associated with picking as well as in her responsibility for the employment of behavioral techniques. The patient continued in behavioral treatment in excess of 1 year, with consequent tapering of fluoxetine. She underwent instruction in relapse prevention and was much improved at 6-month follow-up sessions, which continued for 4 years. Remaining episodes and acute exacerbations were treated as needed by a combination of pharmacotherapy, brief behavioral treatment, and psychodynamic interventions.

The above case example is not intended as a standard recipe, but rather as an illustration of how the use of various mutually facilitating behavioral interventions can be effective, either alone or in combination with pharmacotherapy and psychodynamic understanding, for treating a variety of compulsive SIBs.

# References

Aleksandrowicz MK, Mares AJ: Trichotillomania and trichobezoar in an infant: psychological factors underlying this symptom. J Am Acad Child Psychiatry 17:533–539, 1978

Altman K, Grahs C, Friman PC: Treatment of unobserved trichotillomania by attention reflection and punishment of an apparent covariant. J Behav Ther Exp Psychiatry 13:337–341, 1982

Altman K, Haavik S, Cook W: Punishment of self-injurious behavior in natural settings using contingent aromatic ammonia. Behav Res Ther 16:85–96, 1978

Aronowitz BR, Hollander E: Treating the treatment-resistant patient, in Focus on Obsessive-Compulsive Spectrum Disorders. Edited by Den Boer JA, Westenberg HGM. Amsterdam, the Netherlands, Syn-Thesis, 1997, pp 151–168

Aronowitz BR, Josephson S: Behavioral treatment of obsessive-compulsive spectrum disorders, in Symposium: Obsessive-Compulsive and Related Disorders. New York, The Mount Sinai Medical Center, 1996

Azrin NH, Nunn RG: Habit reversal: a method of eliminating nervous habits and tics. Behav Res Ther 11:619–628, 1973

Azrin NH, Nunn RG, Frantz SE: Habit reversal vs. negative practice treatment of nailbiting. Behav Res Ther 18:281–285, 1980a

Azrin NH, Nunn RG, Frantz SE: Treatment of hair pulling: a comparison study of habit reversal and negative practice training. J Behav Ther Exp Psychiatry 11:13–20, 1980b

Barabasz M: Trichotillomania: a new treatment. Int J Clin Exp Hypn 34:146–154, 1987

Barmann BC, Vitali DL: Facial screening to eliminate trichotillomania in developmentally disabled persons. Behav Ther 13:735–742, 1982

Barrett RP, Shapiro ES: Treatment of stereotyped hair pulling with overcorrection: a case study with long-term follow-up. J Behav Ther Exp Psychiatry 11:317–320, 1980

Barrios BA: Cue-controlled relaxation in reduction of chronic nervous habits. Psychol Rep 41:703–706, 1977

Bayer CA: Self-monitoring and mild aversion treatment of trichotillomania. J Behav Ther Exp Psychiatry 3:139–141, 1972

Bernard ME, Kratochwill TR, Keefauver LW: The effects of rational-emotive therapy and self-instructional training on chronic hair pulling. Cognitive Therapy and Research 7:273–280, 1983

Bornstein PH, Rychtarik RG: Multi-component behavioral treatment of trichotillomania: a case study. Behav Res Ther 16:217–220, 1978

Bornstein PH, Rychtarik RG, McFall ME, et al: Hypnobehavioral treatment of chronic nailbiting. Int J Clin Exp Hypn 28:208–217, 1980

Buxbaum E: Hair pulling and fetishism. Psychoanal Study Child 15:243–260, 1960

Cautela JR: Covert sensitization. Psychol Rep 20:459–468, 1967

Christenson GA, Ristvedt SL, McKenzie TB: Identification of trichotillomania cue profiles. Behav Res Ther 31:315–320, 1993

Connors R: Self-injury in trauma survivors, 2: levels of clinical response. Am J Orthopsychiatry 66:207–216, 1996

Cordle CJ, Long CC: The use of operant self-control procedures in the treatment of compulsive hair pulling. J Behav Ther Exp Psychiatry 11:127–130, 1980

Corte HE, Wolf MM, Locke BJ: A comparison of procedures for eliminating self-injurious behavior of retarded adolescents. J Appl Behav Anal 4:201–213, 1971

Daniels LK: Rapid extinction of nail biting by covert sensitization. J Behav Ther Exp Psychiatry 5:91–92, 1974

Davidson AM, Denney DR, Elliot CH: Suppression and substitution in the treatment of nailbiting. Behav Res Ther 18:1–9, 1980

De Luca RV, Holborn WS: A comparison of relaxation training and competing response training to eliminate hair pulling and nail biting. J Behav Ther Exp Psychiatry 15:67–70, 1984

Derby KM, Fisher WW, Piazza CC: The effects of contingent and noncontingent attention on self-injury and self-restraint. J Appl Behav Anal 29:107–110, 1996

Epstein LH, Peterson GI: The control of undesired behavior by self-imposed contingencies. Behav Ther 4:91–95, 1973

Evans B: A case of trichotillomania in a child treated in a home token program. J Behav Ther Exp Psychiatry 7:197–198, 1976

Fenichel O: The Psychoanalytic Theory of Neuroses. New York, WW Norton and Company, 1945

Finney JW, Rapoff MA, Hall CL, et al: Replication and social validation of habit reversal treatment for tics. Behav Ther 14:116–127, 1983

Fisher WW, Grace NC, Murphy C: Further analysis of the relationship between self-injury and self-restraint. J Appl Behav Anal 29:103–106, 1996

Forehand R, King HE: Pre-school children's non-compliance: effect of short term behavior therapy. Journal of Community Psychology 2:42–44, 1974

Foxx RM, Bechtel DR: Overcorrection, in Progressive Behavior Modification, Vol 13. Edited by Hersen M, Eisler RJ, and Miller PJ. New York, Academic, 1982, pp 277–288

Friman PC, Finney JW, Christophersen ER: Behavioral treatment of trichotillomania: an evaluative review. Behav Ther 15:249–265, 1984

Friman PC, Lucas CP: Behavioral treatment for autism. J Am Acad Child Adolesc Psychiatry 33:1349–1350, 1994

Fruensgaard K: Psychotherapy and neurotic excoriations. Int J Dermatol 30:262–265, 1991a

Fruensgaard K: Psychotherapeutic strategy and neurotic excoriations. Int J Dermatol 3:198–203, 1991b

Gardner GG: Hypnotherapy in the management of childhood habit disorders. J Pediatr 92:838–840, 1978

Greenberg HR, Sarner CA: Trichotillomania: symptom and syndrome. Arch Gen Psychiatry 12:482–489, 1965

Greenberg HR: Transactions of a hairpulling symbiosis. Psychiatr Q 43:662–674, 1969

Grace NC, Thompson R, Fisher WW: The treatment of covert self-injury through contingencies and response products. J Appl Behav Anal 29:239–242, 1996

Gross AM, Farrar MJ, Liner D: Reduction of trichotillomania in a retarded cerebral palsied child using overcorrection, facial screening, and differential reinforcement of other behavior. Education and Treatment of Children 5:133–140, 1982

Hallopeau X: Alopecia par grottag: tichomania au trichotillomania. Ann Dermatol Syphil 10:440, 1889

Honigl D, Kriechbaum N, Zidek D, et al: Self-injury behavior. Acta Med Austriaca 24:19–22, 1997

Horan JJ, Hoffman AM, Macri MG, et al: Self-control of chronic fingernail biting. J Behav Ther Exp Psychiatry 5:307–309, 1974

Horne DJ: Behavior therapy for trichotillomamia. Behav Res Ther 15:192–196, 1977

Horne DJ, Wilkinson J: Habit reversal treatment for fingernail biting. Behav Res Ther 18:287–291, 1980

Irwin D: Alopecia, in Emotional Factors in Skin Disease. Edited by Russel BG, Wittkower ED. New York, Paul Hoeber, 1953

Keuthen N, Aronowitz BR, Wilhelm S, et al: Behavior therapy of trichotillomania, in Trichotillomania. Edited by Stein DJ, Christensen G, Hollander E. Washington, DC, American Psychiatric Press, 1999, pp 147–166

Koblenzer CS: Successful treatment of a chronic and disabling dermatosis by psychotherapy: a case report and discussion. J Am Acad Dermatol 115:390–393, 1986

Koblenzer CS: Psychoanalytic perspectives on trichotillomania, in Trichotillomania. Edited by Stein DJ, Christensen G, Hollander E. Washington, DC, American Psychiatric Press, 1999, pp 125–146

Krishnan KRR, Davidson JRT, Guajardo C: Trichotillomania: a review. Compr Psychiatry 26:123–128, 1985

Ladouceur R: Habit reversal treatment: learning an incompatible response or increasing the subject's awareness? Behav Res Ther 17:313–316, 1979

Langford WS: Disturbance in mother–infant relationship leading to apathy, extranutritional sucking, and hairball, in Emotional Problems of Early Childhood. Edited by Caplan G. New York, Basic Books, 1955, pp 57–86

Levine B: Treatment of trichotillomania by covert sensitization. J Behav Ther Exp Psychiatry 7:75–76, 1976

MacNeil J, Thomas MR: The treatment of obsessive compulsive hair pulling by behavioral and cognitive contingency manipulation. J Behav Ther Exp Psychiatry 7:391–392, 1976

Mannino FV, Delgado RA: Trichotillomania in children: a review. Am J Psychiatry 126:505–511, 1969

Masserman J: Dynamic Psychotherapy. Philadelphia, WB Saunders, 1955

Massong SR, Edwards RP, Range-Sitton L, et al: A case of trichotillomania in a three-year-old treated by response prevention. J Behav Ther Exp Psychiatry 11:223–225, 1980

Mastellone M: Aversion therapy: a new use for the old rubber band. J Behav Ther Exp Psychiatry 5:311–312, 1974

Matson JL, Stephens RM, Smith C: Treatment of self-injurious behavior with over-correction. J Ment Defic Res 22:175–178, 1978

McLaughlin JG, Nay WR: Treatment of trichotillomania using positive coverants and response cost: a case report. Behav Ther 6:87–91, 1975

Meade LS: Covert positive reinforcement in treatment of nailbiting. Dissertation Abstracts International 39:3530–3531, 1979

Meichenbaum DH: Cognitive modification of test anxious college students. J Consult Clin Psychol 39:370–380, 1972

Miltenberger RG, Fuqua RW: A comparison of contingent vs non-contingent competing response practice in the treatment of nervous habits. J Behav Ther Exp Psychiatry 16:195–200, 1985

Miltenberger RG, Fuqua RW, McKinley T: Habit reversal: replication and component analysis. Behav Ther 16:39–50, 1985

Monroe JT Jr, Abse DW: The psychopathology of trichotillomania and trichophagy. Psychiatry 26:95–104, 1963

Norton LA: Self-induced trauma to the nails. Cutis 40:223–227, 1987

Obermayer ME: Psychocutaneous Medicine. Springfield, IL, Charles C Thomas, 1955

Oguchi T, Miura S: Trichotillomania: its psychopathological aspect. Compr Psychiatry 18:177–182, 1977

Ollendick TH: Self-monitoring and self-administered overcorrection: the modification of nervous tics in children. Behav Mod 5:75–84, 1981

O'Reilly MF: Assessment and treatment of episodic self-injury: a case study. Res Dev Disabil 17:349–361, 1996

Ottens AJ: Multifaceted treatment of compulsive hair-pulling. J Behav Ther Exp Psychiatry 12:77–80, 1981

Ottens AJ: A cognitive-behavioral modification treatment of trichotillomania. J Am Coll Health 31:78–81, 1982

Paquin MJ: The treatment of a nail-biting compulsion by covert sensitization in a poorly motivated client. J Behav Ther Exp Psychiatry 8:181–183, 1977

Risch CR, Ferguson JM: Behavioral treatment of skin disorders, in The Comprehensive Handbook of Behavioral Medicine, Vol. 2. Edited by Ferguson JM, Taylor CB. New York, Spectrum, 1981, pp 263–278

Ristvedt SL, Christenson GA: The use of pharmacologic pain sensitization in the treatment of repetitive hair-pulling. Behav Res Ther 34:647–648, 1996

Rosenbaum MS: Treating hair pulling in a 7-year-old male: modified habit reversal for use in pediatric settings. Dev Behav Pediatr 3:241–243, 1982

Rosenbaum MS, Ayllon T: The habit reversal technique in treating trichotillomania. Behav Ther 12:473–481, 1981

Ross JA: The use of contingency contracting in controlling adult nailbiting. J Behav Ther Exp Psychiatry 5:105–106, 1974

Rothbaum BO: Brief clinical reports: the behavioral treatment of trichotillomania. Behav Psychother 20:85–90, 1992

Rothbaum BO, Ninan P: Treatment of trichotillomania: behavior therapy versus clomipramine. Presented at the Association for the Advancement of Behavior Therapy Annual Convention, Boston, MA, November 1992

Rothbaum BO, Shaw L, Morris R, et al: The prevalence of trichotillomania in a college freshman population. J Clin Psychiatry 54:72–73, 1993

Saper B: A report on behavior therapy with outpatient clinic patients. Psychiatr Q 45:209–215, 1971

Scott MJ Jr, Scott MJ III: Dermatophagia: "wolf-biter." Cutis 59:19–20, 1997

Seitz PFD: Dynamically oriented brief psychotherapy: psychocutaneous excoriation syndromes. Psychosom Med 15:200–213, 1953

Singh AN, Maguire J: Trichotillomania and incest. Br J Psychiatry 155:108–110, 1989

Smith FH: Effects of a treatment for nail-biting (abstract). Dissertations Abstracts International 39:789, 1978

Stabler B, Warren AB: Behavioral contracting in treating trichotillomania: a case note. Psychol Rep 34:293–301, 1974

Steck WD: The clinical evaluation of pathologic hair loss. Cutis 24:293–301, 1979

Stevens MJ: Behavioral treatment of trichotillomania. Psychol Rep 55:987–990, 1984

Tarnowski KJ, Rosen LA, McGrath ML, et al: A modified habit reversal procedure in a recalcitrant case of trichotillomania. J Behav Ther Exp Psychiatry 18:157–163, 1987

Taylor JG: A behavioral interpretation of obsessive-compulsive neurosis. Behav Res Ther 1:237–244, 1963

Vitulano LA, King RA, Scahill L, et al: Behavioral treatment of children and adolescents with trichotillomania. J Am Acad Child Adolesc Psychiatry 31:139–146, 1992

Welkowitz LA, Held JL, Held AL, et al: Management of neurotic scratching with behavioral therapy. J Am Acad Dermatol 21:802–804, 1989

Winchel R: Trichotillomania: presentation and treatment. Psychiatr Ann 22:84–89, 1992

Wolfsohn D, Barling J: From external to self-control: behavioral treatment of trichotillomania in an eleven-year-old girl. Psychol Rep 42:1171–1174, 1978

Wolpe J: The Practice of Behavior Therapy. New York, Pergamon, 1973

Zaidens SH: Self-inflicted dermatoses and their psychodynamics. J Nerve Ment Dis 113:395–404, 1951

Zaidens SH: Self-induced dermatoses: psychodynamics and treatment. Skin 3:135–143, 1964

# CHAPTER 6

# Impulsive Self-Injurious Behaviors
## *Neurobiology and Psychopharmacology*

Robert Grossman, M.D.
Larry Siever, M.D.

## Background and Phenomenology

Impulsive self-injurious behavior (SIB) is an explicit part of the DSM-IV (American Psychiatric Association 1994) diagnostic criteria for borderline personality disorder (BPD) and impulse control disorder not otherwise specified. Impulsive SIB is also quite frequently seen in antisocial personality disorder, eating disorders, dissociative disorders, and occasionally in depressive disorders and posttraumatic stress disorder; when it occurs in these latter disorders it may be more common in patients with comorbid Axis II pathology. In practice, the clinician most frequently encounters problematic impulsive SIB in patients with BPD. Approximately 75% of patients with a diagnosis of BPD engage in impulsive SIB (Clarkin et al. 1983), and it is a frequent reason for emergency room visits and hospitalization in the BPD population (Koenigsberg 1982). Impulsive SIB is resistant to treatment and is often extremely disturbing to the friends and family members of the patient, resulting in marked social estrangement (Grunebaum and Klerman 1967; Ross and McKay 1979).

Impulsive SIB is not a homogeneous phenomenon and may be associated with various subjective experiences and accompanying motivations. The typical progression of a patient's internal state surrounding an episode of impulsive SIB involves a precipitating event (typically perceived rejection); escalating dysphoria; attempts to forestall the self-injury; the self-injurious act itself; and the ensuing relief (Leibenluft et al. 1987). The dysphoric feelings sometimes cannot be expressed by the patient but when accessible may be fear, shame, anger, loneliness, and panic. A significant number of patients describe escalating dissociative experiences such as feeling numb, empty, or dead immediately before the injurious act. One-half to three-fourths of BPD patients engaging in impulsive SIB claim marked anesthesia during the event (A.R. Gardner and Gardner 1975; Leibenluft et al. 1987; Roy 1978). The "relief" that many chronic impulsive SIB patients experience after the act may relate to decreased feelings of dissociation, concrete atonement for being bad, or the replacement of physical for emotional pain. Although it is maladaptive, impulsive SIB can be viewed as a form of self-soothing or survival, one that is so effective and ingrained that treatment or substituting other means of self-regulation may be very difficult.

## Challenges of Research and Neurobiologic Considerations

### Heterogeneity of Impulsive Self-Injurious Behavior and Related Behaviors

As a behavior with various associated precipitants and accompanying subjective experiences, impulsive SIB is clearly a heterogeneous phenomenon. There is also diagnostic heterogeneity of individuals engaging in impulsive SIB. Researchers have begun to pursue consistent neurobiologic associations that transcend diagnostic and phenomenologic categorizations. A uniform neurobiology of such a behavior, however, may not exist. It may instead be reasonable to expect that impulsive SIB could be associated with various neurobiologic and functional alterations.

### Paucity of Data

Currently, very few neurobiologic and treatment studies specifically of impulsive SIB are available. If, however, the disorder is viewed as a behavior associated with other behaviors such as increased impulsivity, aggression, dissociation, or suicide, it is possible to cast a wider net in our exploration. This chapter discusses both impulsive SIB and associated behaviors.

### Associated Behaviors

As the nosology indicates, impulsive SIB has an element of impulsivity. However, a fair number of patients plan these behaviors (e.g., go to the store and buy razors or wait until they can be in the bathroom or other area undisturbed). As DSM-IV states

> The essential feature of Impulse Control Disorders is the failure to resist an impulse, drive, or temptation to perform an act that is harmful to the person or to others...the individual feels an increasing sense of tension or arousal before committing the act and then experiences pleasure, gratification, or relief at the time of committing the act. (p. 609)

Therefore, impulsive acts such as SIB, gambling, and others may involve a component of planning. Impulsivity is a personality characteristic that can be measured through various self-reported and clinician ratings, and its neurobiologic correlates have been studied fairly extensively.

The act of physically injuring oneself can also be viewed as an aggressive behavior and may be more common among aggressive individuals. Aggressive behaviors may be directed toward the self or toward others. Suicide attempts may be viewed as an example of self-directed aggression, whereas homicidality or physical attacks against others are considered to be types of outward-directed aggression. Aggression, like impulsivity, can be quantified and studied in relation to various neurobiologic, metabolic, genetic, and other measures and has also been studied extensively.

By definition, impulsive SIB is without suicidal intent, yet approximately 60% of BPD subjects engaging in this behavior have a history of one or more true suicide attempts. Neurobiologic studies, as is discussed later in the chapter, have found various associations with attempted and completed suicide. Therefore, studies in this area should control for history of past suicide attempts. This is difficult, however, and few studies have been able to do so.

Another question is whether biologic findings associated with impulsive SIB are to be viewed as "trait" or "state" variables or a particular combination of the two. *Trait variables* are enduring physiologic variables and as such are constant over time and therefore found in association with the behavioral measure regardless of how temporally related the behavioral event and biologic measure are. Trait variables would be present at a higher rate in individuals engaging in impulsive SIB regardless of whether the assessment occurred before, during, or after the act. *State variables*, however, are viewed as temporally related to the independent variable (in this case, impulsive SIB) and are thought to be reflective of the biologic state of the individual at the time of the behavior.

Impulsive SIB is known to be associated with psychologic measures of impulsivity and aggression, yet the susceptibility to impulsive acts appears to be a heritable trait, associated with biologic correlates that are sta-

**Table 6–1.** Challenges of research on impulsive self-injurious behavior

Heterogeneity of diagnostic, phenomenologic, and precipitating states in the impulsive self-injurious behavior population

Relatively few neurobiologic studies specifically of impulsive self-injurious behavior available to serve as pilot data for future directions in research

State versus trait aspects of neurobiology need to be differentiated

Past/current suicidality difficult to control for

Neurobiologic/physiologic alterations may result from physical impact of self-injurious act

ble over time and not necessarily temporally related to the impulsive/ aggressive acts themselves (Coccarro et al. 1993). The marked strong affects or intense dissociation experienced by most individuals immediately before impulsive SIB usually is transient (although reoccurring) and could reasonably be assumed to be associated with biologic state variables. Yet from a broader perspective, affective dysregulation or dissociation could be traits. In most cases the patient clearly reports that the behavior was engaged in to bring about a state change in his or her thought patterns or emotional experience. These state variables would be hypothesized to become less pronounced the longer one waits to measure them after the self-injurious event.

One must further consider the physiologic and neurobiologic effects occurring with tissue damage during such extreme acts as cutting or burning oneself. Presumably these impulsive SIB–induced changes would be most pronounced immediately following the episode and decay with time. These state-dependent, time-related effects are difficult to study using retrospective designs. Only associations, not cause–effect relationships can be ascertained. Prospective studies, however, are more difficult because they require a greater sample size and repeated assessments, take longer to complete, and involve the ethical responsibility of intervention in order to both prevent the behaviors and teach alternative practices and modulatory techniques to help the patient decrease these behaviors. Table 6–1 summarizes the dilemmas involved in the neurobiologic study of impulsive SIB.

## Neurobiologic Studies and Related Phenomena

Very few neurobiologic studies of impulsive SIB have been made. Findings from these few studies are discussed in depth and supplemented with relevant discussion of neurobiologic studies of psychologic measures associated with impulsive SIB, namely impulsivity, aggression, dissociation, and suicide.

## Serotonergic Pathways

### Impulsive Aggression and Serotonergic Studies

The first studies linking impulsive-aggressive behavior with serotonin function in humans used measurement of cerebrospinal fluid (CSF) 5-hydroxyindolacetic acid (5-HIAA), the primary metabolite of serotonin. In depressed patients, CSF 5-HIAA concentration was inversely related to violent/lethal suicidal behavior (Asberg et al. 1976). Among male naval recruits meeting DSM-III (American Psychiatric Association 1980) criteria for BPD, inverse correlations were reported between CSF 5-HIAA and both lifetime history of aggression (G.L. Brown et al. 1979) and psychopathic deviance on the Minnesota Multiphasic Personality Inventory (G.L. Brown et al. 1982). CSF 5-HIAA was significantly lower among impulsive violent offenders and arsonists than among premeditated violent offenders (Linnoila et al. 1983), suggesting that decreased serotonin function correlates more specifically with impulsive-aggressive behavior than with violence per se. Not all studies have found significant correlations. In a sample of women with severe BPD, no correlation was found between lifetime history of aggression and CSF 5-HIAA (D.L. Gardner et al. 1990), nor was a correlation found in another study of 24 subjects with personality disorder (Coccaro et al. 1997b).

Other studies have assessed serotonergic activity using neuropharmacologic challenges. One of the first studies reported that in men with depression and personality disorder, aggression and history of suicide attempts were inversely related to the prolactin response to fenfluramine (Coccaro et al. 1989). Fenfluramine is both a serotonin releasing agent and a reuptake inhibitor that has been postulated to assess both pre- and postsynaptic serotonin activity, or net serotonergic function. Among all subjects with personality disorders, the group of individuals with anger dyscontrol, impulsivity, and self-damaging behavior had a significantly lower prolactin response to fenfluramine than subjects without these criteria (Coccaro et al. 1989). Other studies have confirmed these findings in nondepressed suicidal individuals (Siever and Trestman 1993) and another group of subjects with personality disorder (Coccaro et al. 1997b). Agents with serotonin receptor subtype specificity have also been used in challenge paradigms. Ipsapirone is a selective serotonin-1A agonist thought to produce changes in cortisol level secondary to activation of postsynaptic hypothalamic receptors and changes in body temperature through activation of presynaptic somatodendritic autoreceptors (Lesch et al. 1990a, 1990b). In an interesting pilot study, cortisol response to ipsapirone was inversely correlated at a trend level with Buss-Durkee Hostility Inventory verbal assault, whereas temperature response was inversely correlated with Brown-Goodwin Assault–Revised aggression score (Coccaro et al. 1995). Using buspirone, another selective serotonin-1A agonist, decreased prolactin response was found to correlate with self-assessed irritability (Coccaro et al. 1990b).

Siever and colleagues recently assessed serotonin function in 97 patients with DSM-III personality disorders using a fenfluramine challenge. Of these patients, 87 also participated in a placebo arm of the study. A three-level variable was constructed as a composite of suicide attempts and tissue damage with values from 0 to 2 (0 = those with neither suicide attempts nor tissue-damaging acts; 1 = those with either suicide attempts or impulsive SIB; and 2 = those with a history of both behaviors); this was done to quantify the extent of self-directed aggression (of which we viewed suicide attempts and impulsive SIB as two manifestations) and because in total only a few of the patients who engaged in impulsive SIB did not have a history of suicide attempts. Among the men, the composite self-directed aggression score was inversely related to prolactin response—that is, decreased serotonergic activity was associated with increased levels of self-directed aggression. Fewer women were studied and their response to fenfluramine was more variable and not statistically significant (New et al. 1997).

Serotonergic functioning has also been assessed through assay of specific serotonin receptors and transporters on circulating platelets and in the brain. Significant evidence exists that platelet receptor data reflects analogous structures in the brain. Increased numbers of platelet serotonin-2A binding sites have been reported in suicide attempters (Biegon et al. 1990). In patients who successfully committed suicide, increased numbers of serotonin-2A binding sites were found posthumously in the cortex and amygdala compared with those found in normal controls (Arora and Meltzer 1989; Arango et al. 1990). Using $^{125}$I-LSD, number and affinity of serotonin-2A binding sites on platelets was directly correlated with personality disordered subjects' self-reports of aggressive tendencies (Coccaro et al. 1997b). Platelet studies have reported decreased serotonin uptake (using tritiated imipramine binding) in aggressive adults (C.S. Brown et al. 1989) and children with conduct disorder (Stoff et al. 1987). Serotonin uptake was found to have an inverse correlation with impulsivity scores in aggressive men (C.S. Brown et al. 1989). Tritiated paroxetine, a more sensitive and selective radioligand for the serotonin transporter, has been recently used in a study reporting an inverse correlation between number of serotonin transporter sites and lifetime history of aggression (Coccaro et al. 1996).

One study (Simeon et al. 1992) compared platelet imipramine binding ($B_{max}$), affinity ($K_d$), and CSF 5-HIAA levels in 26 patients with personality disorder and impulsive SIB with those in 26 matched control subjects with personality disorder who did not engage in impulsive SIB. Interestingly, the groups were not significantly different from each other on any of the three measures of serotonin function. Furthermore, impulsivity (as measured by a subscale of the Schedule for Interviewing Borderlines that included behaviors such as gambling, overspending, promiscuity, overeating, and oversleeping) was not significantly different between groups. The self-mutilators, however, were more aggressive. Among self-mutilators, a significant inverse correlation was found between $B_{max}$ level and severity of self-injury. The authors hypothesized that greater aggression, in combination with poor impulse control, is more likely to take the form of impulsive SIB rather than the less-aggressive impulsive behaviors assessed by the Schedule for Interviewing Borderlines (Simeon et al. 1992).

### Evidence for Heritability of Impulsive Aggression as Related to Serotonin Function

A blunted prolactin response to fenfluramine in personality-disordered probands has been reported to be a better predictor of impulsivity in their relatives than impulsive traits themselves (Coccaro et al. 1997a). Reduced serotonergic function may thus be the primary familially transmitted trait that may interact with environmental stressors such as trauma and result in impulsive-aggressive behaviors. Family history studies have found that first-degree relatives of patients with histories of violent behavior have a higher incidence of violent behavior (Bach-Y-Rita et al. 1971; Maletsky 1973).

Further evidence for the heritability of impulsive aggression comes from twin studies in children, adolescents, and adults. The results have been quite variable and can be partly explained by differences in measures used in the various studies. Four adult studies found heritability estimates with a range of 41%–72% (Cates et al. 1993; Coccaro et al. 1993; Rushton et al. 1986; Tellegen et al. 1988). In general, heritability of impulsive aggression appears to increase and become more robust with increasing age. A possible explanation is that a non–impulsive-aggressive adopting family serves to modulate such behavior in a child with an impulsive-aggressive genotype. With the passage of time and aging of the individual, the environment's ability to curb such behavior decreases.

Molecular genetic techniques are providing further data on the relationship between altered serotonergic functioning and impulsivity/aggression. The major serotonin degrading enzyme is monoamine oxidase type A (MAOA). Using transgene insertion, a knockout mouse line lacking MAOA was produced. These mice displayed increased aggressive behavior associated with increased brain serotonin concentrations (Cases et al. 1995). In a family in which some members had a point mutation in the gene encoding for MAOA, the mutation was associated with increased aggressiveness (Brunner et al. 1993). These findings may indicate that bimodal effects of either low or high serotonergic activity are associated with aggression. Compensation by other involved neurotransmitters or decreased sensitivity of postsynaptic serotonin receptors could theoretically result in a phenotype (aggression) usually associated with decreased serotonin activity.

Another genetic mutant mouse was engineered for deletion of the serotonin-1B receptor. These serotonin-1B receptor–lacking mice showed a more rapid and fierce attack on intruding mice (resident–intruder paradigm) than did the unaltered (wild type) mice (Saudou et al. 1994). Other examples of increased aggression in mice with genetic alterations affecting serotonergic activity include the overexpression of transforming growth factor alpha (decreased serotonin in the CSF) (Hilakivi-Clarke et al. 1995) and heterozygous calcium calmodulin–dependent protein kinase II (reduced serotonin release from the raphe nuclei) (Chen et al. 1994).

Tryptophan hydroxylase (TPH) is the rate-regulating enzyme in the formation of serotonin. In molecular genetic studies in humans, it was found that within Finnish violent criminal offenders with alcoholic histories, an allelic variant of TPH is associated with suicide attempts (Nielsen et al. 1994). In a pilot study, an increase in the LL allele of TPH was associated with increased levels of hostility (New et al. 1998). Two allelic variants of the serotonin transporter gene have been recently identified, one of which was found to be significantly associated with increased angry hostility and impulsiveness (Lesch et al. 1996).

### Functional Neuroimaging

The orbitofrontal cortex is believed to be important in the modulation of impulsive aggression. This area of the brain receives rich serotonergic enervation from the dorsal raphe nucleus. Depressed suicidal patients, compared with depressed control subjects, were found to show decreased fenfluramine-induced metabolic activation of frontal glucose metabolism (Mann et al. 1996). Among a mixed group of subjects with personality disorder, glucose metabolism in the cerebral cortex was found to be inversely correlated with a life history of aggressive impulse difficulties (Goyer et al. 1994).

In summary, various means of assessing serotonin function, including challenge studies, receptor and transporter assays, and functional neuroimaging, have found a strong correlation between impulsivity, aggression, suicidality, and serotonin function. Specifically, decreased serotonin function is associated with increased impulsivity, increased aggression and increased suicidality. Other studies, however, have failed to show differences in serotonin function between self-injurious and non-self-injurious subjects with personality disorder.

## The Endogenous Opioid System

Several aspects of the phenomenology associated with impulsive SIB in BPD patients suggest possible involvement of the endogenous opioid system (EOS). As previously stated, one-half to three-fourths of BPD patients engaging in impulsive SIB claim marked anesthesia during the event (A.R. Gardner et al. 1975; Leibenluft et al. 1987; Roy 1978). Affective states may also alter pain perception. Patients with BPD frequently have comorbid Axis I disorders (Widiger and Rogers 1989) associated with diminished pain responsiveness. These include major depression, eating disorders, and posttraumatic stress disorder (van der Kolk et al. 1989). Abundant evidence indicates EOS involvement in pain perception, particularly in stress-induced analgesia (Amir et al. 1980; Madden et al. 1977).

Several researchers have postulated that enhanced brain opioid activity may underlie SIB in certain individuals (R.P. Barrett et al. 1989; Bernstein et al 1987; Davidson et al. 1983; Herman 1990; Herman et al. 1987; Richardson and Zaleski 1983; Sandman et al. 1983; Sandyk 1985). The two most prominent hypotheses to account for SIB in humans are the addiction hypothesis (Richardson and Zaleski 1983; Sandman et al. 1983) and the pain hypothesis (Barron and Sandman 1985). The addiction hypothesis suggests that there exists an essentially normal EOS that has been chronically overstimulated by frequent SIB for the purpose of relieving dysphoria. The individual develops a tolerance to the outpouring of endogenous opioids, cyclically suffers a withdrawal reaction, and is driven to further EOS stimulation by means of impulsive SIB (Coid et al. 1983; Leibenluft et al. 1987; Richardson and Zaleski 1983, 1986; Sandman et al. 1987). The pain hypothesis suggests a constitutional abnormality in the EOS that is unmasked by the environment such that pain sensitivity is diminished. This may involve a lack of negative feedback in the EOS and/or overproduction of endogenous opioids. This heightened opiatergic tone could eventually lead to dysphoric experiences of numbness and dissociation. SIB may present a stimulus that breaks through a self-alienating dissociative state, brought on by environmental and/or intrapsychic stressors, and thereby allows the self-injurer to feel again.

Russ et al. (1993) reported that pain ratings during a cold pressor test (submerging the hand and/or forearm in an ice water bath) were significantly lower in patients with BPD who reported anesthesia during impulsive SIB than in similar patients who reported feeling pain and in normal control subjects. BPD subjects who engaged in impulsive SIB were also less able to differentiate among various intensities of painful stimuli (Russ et al. 1992). The relative analgesia of the first group, however, may not be EOS mediated, because this analgesia was not reversed by the opioid receptor antagonist naloxone (Russ et al. 1994). The authors suggested, however, that the cold pressor test may not be an adequate stimulus for EOS activation. Thus, a role for the EOS in SIB is not ruled out.

The relief of dysphoria, perhaps the most common goal of impulsive SIB, may involve the EOS. Typically, impulsive SIB is followed in minutes to hours by cessation of dissociative symptoms and a feeling of relief (Favazza and Conterio 1989; D.L. Gardner and Cowdry 1985; Grunebaum and Klerman 1967). This effect has been noted in laboratory cold pressor pain tests, which found that those BPD individuals who report pain during SIB indicated no change in affective state after the painful stimulus, whereas BPD individuals with analgesia during impulsive SIB indicated improvement in areas of depression, anxiety, anger, and confusion (Russ et al. 1992). Endogenous opioids may be involved in mood regulation, particularly under conditions of social stress (Panksepp et al. 1978).

In another study, plasma corticotropin (adrenocorticotropic hormone, ACTH), N-terminal lipotropin, C-terminal lipotropin (β-endorphin–like immunoreactivity), and met-enkephalin levels were measured in 10 drug-free patients with BPD diagnosed using DSM-III criteria. Subjects had engaged in at least three episodes of SIB, at least two of which were carried out without pain, followed by relief of tension or dysphoria. Compared with that found in normal control subjects, the plasma met-enkephalin concentration in these patients was significantly higher. No group differences were found for other neuropeptides (Coid et al. 1983). These results, however, need to be viewed cautiously because SIB per se can cause elevations in plasma endogenous opiates. Genetically manipulated lines of mice with a deficiency in pre-proenkephalin (and enkephalin) showed increased aggression in the resident–intruder paradigm (Konig et al. 1996).

## Noradrenergic and Other Pathways

Animal data are consistent with the view that central noradrenergic function regulates the organism's level of arousal and responsiveness to environmental stimuli (Aston-Jones and Bloom 1981; Rasmussen et al. 1986). Therefore, increased noradrenergic activity is associated with increased readiness to respond to environmental stimuli, aversive or not. The number of shock-induced aggressive episodes in rodents has been found to directly correlate with increased noradrenergic function in the brain (Stolk et al. 1974). Conversely, pharmacologic agents that enhance central noradrenergic function (such as tricyclic antidepressants [TCAs] and monoamine oxidase inhibitors [MAOIs]) increases shock-induced fighting in rodents (Eichelman and Barchas 1975).

A primary metabolite of norepinephrine is 3-methoxy-4-hydroxyphenylglycol (MHPG). Some studies in humans have found a direct correlation between CSF levels of MHPG with extroversion (Roy et al. 1989) and history of impulsive aggression (G.L. Brown et al. 1979), whereas others have not (D.L. Gardner et al. 1990; Linnoila et al. 1983). Siever and Trestman (1993) reported a positive correlation between plasma norepinephrine and self-reported impulsivity in men with personality disorder. Clonidine, an $\alpha_2$ agonist, has been used as a probe of noradrenergic function by measuring growth hormone response to intravenous challenge. Among groups of healthy male volunteers, men with major affective disorders, and men with personality disorders, the growth hormone response to clonidine challenge was found to positively correlate with the Irritability subscale score of the Buss-Durkee Hostility Inventory, but not with the Assault subscale (Coccaro et al. 1991).

The relationship between dopamine and impulsive aggression is unclear. In a sample of women with severe BPD, no correlation was found between lifetime history of aggression and CSF levels of the dopamine metabolite homovanillic acid (HVA) (D.L. Gardner et al. 1990). Studies of other populations did not find a relationship between CSF HVA levels and aggression (G.L. Brown et al. 1979; Virkkunen et al. 1987).

As discussed previously, impulsive SIB may be used to regulate mood. The acetylcholinesterase inhibitor physostigmine has been used as a challenge agent to investigate acute effects on mood in patients with personality disorder and in healthy volunteers. Compared with other subjects with personality disorders, patients with BPD experienced greater mood effects during the challenge that positively correlated with the number of affective instability traits. However, mood effects that occurred during the challenge were not significantly correlated with impulsive-aggressive traits (Steinberg et al. 1997).

## Psychopharmacologic Treatment

No medication for the treatment of impulsive SIB has yet been approved by the U.S. Food and Drug Administration. Furthermore, no double-blind or placebo-controlled studies of medications for the treatment of this disorder have been performed. The few pharmacologic treatment studies specifically for impulsive SIB are reviewed here, in addition to pharmacologic treatment studies suggesting efficacy for symptoms/signs related to impulsive SIB, including impulsivity, aggression, rejection sensitivity, and dissociation.

Patients who engage in impulsive SIB often meet diagnostic criteria for a cluster B personality disorder (usually borderline, antisocial) and/or an eating disorder such as bulimia or anorexia. Forming a therapeutic alliance with the patient and educating him or her about medication side effects, target symptoms, and realistic expectations of treatment response are critical. Pharmacologic treatment of such patients should usually occur in a setting of ongoing psychotherapy because a patient's engagement in impulsive SIB is usually a response to overwhelming emotional experiences in an individual with few or no other means of affect regulation. As discussed in Chapter 1, histories of sexual abuse and other traumatic/chaotic experiences often populate these patients' formative years. The lack of appropriate interpersonal experiences and the attendant conflicts in the areas of trust, self-esteem, mood regulation, and self-soothing cannot be resolved with medication. Rather, appropriate pharmacologic treatment can lessen the intensity of certain experiences and create a more favorable setting for psychotherapy and long-term characterologic/behavioral changes.

Because approximately 60% of the patients engaging in impulsive SIB make an actual suicide attempt at some point in their lives, medications with narrow therapeutic margins or lethality in overdose should only be used with great caution or preferably not at all. Table 6–2 summarizes findings for the pharmacologic agents discussed below.

### Selective Serotonin Reuptake Inhibitors

The utility of selective serotonin reuptake inhibitors (SSRIs) has been investigated in the treatment of impulsive aggression and impulsive SIB. An open-label trial of fluoxetine in two patients with BPD was reported. The maximum decrease in verbal aggression and irritability in these two patients occurred at week 3 while they were receiving 20 mg of fluoxetine. Neither of these subjects was reported to be engaging in impulsive SIB. A decrease in positive effects of the medication occurred, and in both cases fluoxetine was raised to 40 mg but without a return to the briefly observed level of improvement (Coccaro et al. 1990a). Other investigators have observed anti-impulsive effects that are rapidly lost and only partially recoverable through dose increase. In an open-label trial of fluoxetine, Norden (1989) found that 9 of 12 patients were judged to be much or very much

**Table 6–2.** Psychopharmacologic treatment of impulsive self-injurious behavior

| Medication | Target symptoms that may be associated with impulsive SIB* | Remarks |
|---|---|---|
| SSRIs/NSRIs | Impulsivity, depression, anxiety, irritability, aggression | Patients are often sensitive to increased anxiety as a side effect; therefore, start at a lower dose and increase slowly. Clinical response may also occur at a lower dose. Treatment of impulsivity frequently requires a higher dose and clinical effects may be short-lived, which may lead to stepwise increases followed by eventual ineffectiveness. Watch for iatrogenic hypomania/mania. In general, one of the safest and most effective medications in this population. NSRIs (nefazadone and venlafaxine) may theoretically have a greater chance of causing behavioral dyscontrol secondary to noradrenergic activity—*see* tricyclic antidepressants. |
| Mood stabilizers | Mood lability, impulsivity, anxiety | Divalproex sodium may be the best tolerated. Carbamazepine has been associated with possible increase in occurrence of depression. Gabapentin is quite sedating and may help with sleep but may be less effective unless combined with another mood stabilizer. Lithium is often poorly tolerated and is lethal in overdose. |
| Opioid antagonists | Perhaps of highest efficacy in association with history of sexual abuse and analgesia during impulsive SIB | Limited open-label evidence, theoretic possibility of an initial escalation of impulsive SIB if the dysphoria-improving qualities are eliminated by the antagonist. Perhaps more effective in patients reporting analgesia during impulsive SIB. |
| β-Blockers | Impulsivity, aggression, dissociation, hyperarousal | Both antagonists and partial agonists may be used. Propranolol is the most likely to cause orthostasis, and all may cause depression. High doses may decrease switching between alters in dissociative identity disorders. |

**Table 6–2.** Psychopharmacologic treatment of impulsive self-injurious behavior (*continued*)

| Medication | Target symptoms that may be associated with impulsive SIB* | Remarks |
|---|---|---|
| Antipsychotic agents | Aggression, anxiety, experiences of ego disintegration secondary to sensory/input overload | Consider atypical agents, but realize that a medication such as olanzapine may cause significant weight gain with accompanying self-esteem issues. Start with small doses. A certain number of patients with borderline personality disorder will prefer a small dose of a standard neuroleptic, perhaps those with more cognitive disorganization. |
| Benzodiazepines | Overwhelming anxiety, irritability | Use with caution in all patients, and relatively contraindicated if history of past/current substance abuse. Long-acting agents are preferable (clonazepam) and dosing can be either standing or as needed. Disinhibition with increased impulsivity/aggression may occur, especially with shorter-acting agents such as alprazolam. *Cautious use.* |
| Monoamine oxidase inhibitors | Depression, rejection sensitivity | Certainly not a first-line medication. Dangers of drug interactions, hypertensive crises, overdose. Sometimes effective for a very treatment-resistant dysthymia/depression that has not responded to other medications. *Cautious use.* |
| Tricyclic antidepressants | Depression | Lethal in overdose, noradrenergic effects may increase impulsivity and behavioral dyscontrol. *Cautious use.* |

*This is labeled as such because medications in subjects with borderline personality disorder most frequently have global effects, therefore any class of medication may potentially decrease any symptom. This also implies that the effect in a given patient may be different than the medication "class" may indicate—i.e., an "antidepressant" may primarily decrease a patient's anxiety, a "mood stabilizer" may primarily serve to decrease impulsivity, and an SSRI may decrease psychotic symptoms.
*Note.* NSRIs = norepinephrine and serotonin reuptake inhibitors; SSRIs = selective serotonin reuptake inhibitors.

improved after 5–26 weeks. Depression and impulsivity were thought to have improved the most. This report did not comment on impulsive SIB in these subjects, but noted that benefits were still evident after 6 months of treatment. Another group treated five patients with BPD with fluoxetine at a dose of 20–40 mg/day and reported improved functioning and a decrease in dysphoria (Cornelius et al. 1990).

A 12-week open-label trial of 80 mg/day fluoxetine was conducted in 22 outpatients who met diagnostic criteria by clinical assessment for BPD and/or schizotypal personality disorder (4 pure schizotypal) (Markowitz et al. 1991). Of these 22 patients, 13 had comorbid major depression. When analyzing all patients together, a diverse range of symptoms, including psychoticism, seemed to respond. The only subgroup that showed significant improvement was that of the patients with depression. Twelve of the patients in this study, all meeting criteria for BPD, were engaging in approximately four incidents of self-mutilation per week. Self-mutilation was quantified by scoring 12-hour periods as positive if self-mutilation occurred during that interval (regardless of severity or number of times). By the final week of the study, only two patients were still engaged in self-mutilation, at a frequency of less than once per week, resulting in a 97% reduction in the calculated self-mutilation score. Data on dropout and side effects were not clear, but it appears from a later study that approximately 22% of patients were intolerant of fluoxetine side effects (Markowitz et al. 1991).

Other serotonergic agents besides fluoxetine have been studied. In an open-label trial of sertraline at doses of 100–200 mg/day, Kavoussi et al. (1994) treated 11 patients, 8 of whom met diagnostic criteria for BPD. Using the Modified Overt Aggression Scale, significant improvement occurred as measured by the mean aggression and irritability scores at week 8, but impulsive SIB was not assessed. Venlafaxine (a noradrenergic-serotonergic reuptake inhibitor) has also been reported to be effective in an open-label trial of 39 patients with scores of seven or higher on the Gunderson Diagnostic Interview for Borderline Personality Disorder (Markowitz and Wagner 1995). Venlafaxine doses ranged from 200 to 400 mg/day for the 12 weeks of treatment. Statistically significant reductions were reported on all 10 subscales of the Symptom Checklist 90. Furthermore, seven of the patients had been engaging in chronic impulsive SIB at the start of the study, but after 12 weeks of treatment only two patients remained self-injurious. Rates of sexual dysfunction as a medication side effect appeared to be lower than in studies of fluoxetine and sertraline.

It is difficult to make statements about efficacy because these trials were open label, lacked a placebo control (especially given the marked placebo effect commonly observed in BPD patients), used nonblind raters, and in some cases were initiated at the time of hospitalization—a period during which significant improvement would be occurring in most patients with BPD secondary to a structured and safe "holding" environment. In a placebo-controlled trial of fluoxetine treatment at 80 mg/day for 14 weeks in subjects with BPD, a wide variety of symptoms showed marked improvement, including suicidality, depression, anxiety, sleep problems, self-injury, obsessionality, aggression, and psychotic behaviors (Markowitz 1995). More recently, a double-blind placebo-controlled trial of nondepressed patients with personality disorder showed fluoxetine to be effective in decreasing measures of irritability and aggression. SIB was not assessed (Coccaro and Kavoussi 1997).

Side effects from the SSRIs increase with dose and may include decreased libido, anorgasmia, insomnia, agitation, tremulousness, and feelings of depersonalization/derealization (PDR 1996). A significant number of patients are not able to tolerate SSRIs. Others appear not to benefit from them. A series of six cases has been published (two of which were of depressed patients with BPD) in which the patients developed severe obsessive suicidal thoughts that were "more intense, violent, and persistent" during fluoxetine treatment (Teicher et al. 1990). Reportedly, none of these patients had ever experienced a similar state during medication treatment. Such side effects are uncommon, but the treating clinician should be aware of the potential occurrence. SSRIs may also precipitate iatrogenic mania (PDR 1996). This is no small consideration in BPD and impulsive patients, many of whom show strong phenomenologic similarities to and actual comorbidity with bipolar I disorder, bipolar II disorder, and cyclothymia.

In general, however, SSRIs are relatively safe medications that are well tolerated. They are the first-line medications for most patients engaging in impulsive SIB, except those with (comorbid) bipolar disorder. Various studies have demonstrated that patients may not tolerate or show a response to one SSRI even if the dose and duration of treatment appears adequate, but will show a good response to a different SSRI. It is reasonable to expect that all SSRIs would probably show similar efficacy as a whole, but in many cases it is prudent to try another SSRI if the response to one is intolerance of side effects or lack of clinical improvement.

## Mood Stabilizers and Anticonvulsants

Mood stabilizers and anticonvulsants have also been used in the treatment of various symptoms of impulsive individuals, yet no studies have assessed self-injury per se as a target symptom. Interest in these medications primarily grew out of their known efficacy in the treatment of mood swings in bipolar disorder and the aforementioned comorbidity and phenomenologic overlap of bipolar-type disorders with impulsive behaviors and BPD. Lithium was one of the first medications reported to be effective in decreasing mood instability in a diagnostic precursor of BPD, namely unstable character disorder (Rifkin et al. 1972). A trend of decreased anger and suicidal symptoms was reported in a placebo-controlled trial of lithium in a small number of patients with BPD but did not appear to be effective for treatment of depressive symptoms, and a high treatment dropout rate was noted (Links et al. 1990). Lithium has been reported to reduce impulsive aggression in prison inmates in a double-blind placebo-controlled trial (Sheard et al. 1976). Lithium, however, may exacerbate aggression in persons with seizure-associated (ictal and interictal) behavioral dyscontrol (Schiff et al. 1982). Lithium requires plasma level monitoring, causes frequent side effects of tremor and weight gain, and is lethal in overdose.

Controlled studies have found other anticonvulsants, such as carbamazepine, to be effective in the treatment of mood instability and impulsive aggression in disorders other than BPD (E.S. Barrett et al. 1992; Blumer et al. 1988; Kravitz and Fawcett 1987; Mattes 1990). In BPD specifically, a crossover study found that carbamazepine produced a significant decrease in the frequency and severity of irritability and aggressive behavior as well as an improvement in mood and anxiety (Cowdry and Gardner 1988). Although carbamazepine is classified as a mood stabilizer, medication effects were diverse and nonspecific. The authors thought that carbamazepine's mood effect was not antidepressant-like, but rather mood stabilizing (Cowdry and Gardner 1988). Treatment with this agent is not without significant problems. Of the 17 patients who were treated with carbamazepine in this study, three developed melancholia that remitted on discontinuation of the agent (D.L. Gardner and Cowdry 1986). Even if carbamazepine did not cause the melancholia, it certainly appears not to have prevented it. Additionally, of 22 patients treated in the entire series, 6 (27%) developed allergic reactions, 3 of whom required medication discontinuation (Cowdry and Gardner 1988). Other problems with carbamazepine include the rare but potentially lethal occurrence of aplastic anemia (PDR 1996).

An open treatment study of divalproex sodium in 11 outpatients with BPD has been conducted but did not specifically assess for impulsive SIB (Stein et al. 1995). Individuals with current and/or past bipolar disorder were excluded and all study patients were in ongoing psychotherapy at least once per week for a minimum of 8 weeks before beginning medication. Treatment consisted of open-label divalproex sodium for 8 weeks with a target plasma valproate level of between 50 and 100 μg/mL. Psychotherapy was continued for the duration of the trial, and no concurrent medication was given. Weekly clinician ratings were administered, including the Hamilton Depression Scale (Ham-D), the Hamilton Anxiety Scale (Ham-A), and the Overt Aggression Scale–Modified (OAS–M). The Cowdry and Gardner Scale (Cowdry and Gardner 1988) was also administered, which is similar to the Clinician Global Impression scale. This scale rates mood, anxiety, anger, impulsivity, rejection sensitivity, and overall pathology on a scale of 1–7. Of the 11 patients initially entered into the study, 3 dropped out. Of the 8 completers, 4 (50%) were considered treatment responders and were rated "much less" or "less" on overall pathology and mood symptoms. In addition, 3 of 8 patients were responders in terms of improvement in anxiety, anger, impulsivity, and rejection sensitivity. There were changes on subscales of the OAS–M that were greater than 50%. Only one of these, global subjective irritability, reached statistical significance, possibly secondary to large standard deviations and the small number of subjects. This study was limited by being an open trial in a small sample (11 patients) and having a relatively short duration (8 weeks). Although impulsive SIB was not rated, a decrease in anxiety, anger, and rejection sensitivity could possibly result in decreased impulsive SIB. Larger controlled trials of divalproex sodium in BPD were judged to be warranted.

Clinical experience and one recent study have shown once-daily dosing to be effective and well tolerated for affective disorders (Balfour and Bryson 1994). Target plasma valproate levels for treatment of impulsive aggression are probably similar to those used for mood-stabilizing and anti-seizure effects. Some patients, however, may show a clinical response below the usual range of 50 μg/mL, whereas others may require more than 100 μg/mL. Similar to more treatment-refractory bipolar patients, some patients with impulsive aggression or mood lability may benefit from a combination of mood stabilizing agents, but this has not been scientifically studied.

Valproate has several theoretical reasons for its potential efficacy in BPD and other disorders with marked impulsivity (Hollander et al. 1996). Divalproex sodium/valproate has demonstrated efficacy in cyclothymia (Deltito 1993; Jacobsen 1993) and bipolar I and II disorders (Jacobsen 1993; McElroy et al. 1987; Schaff et al. 1993), which have considerable overlap with BPD symptoms. From a dimensional perspective, there are anecdotal reports of divalproex sodium decreasing aggression and impulsivity (Giakas et al. 1990; Hasan et al. 1990; Keck et al. 1992). As a mood stabilizer, divalproex sodium may be better tolerated and safer than carbamazepine.

One mechanism of divalproex sodium action in some individuals may be through a reduction of limbic kindling phenomena. Divalproex sodium may uniquely combine the GABA-ergic antianxiety properties of the benzodiazepines (without the risks of behavioral disinhibition), the serotonergic anti-impulsive/antidepressant properties of the SSRIs (without the risks of agitation or mania), and the mood-stabilizing effects of carbamazepine (without the high incidence of allergic reactions, depression, or aplastic anemia/agranulocytosis).

The most common side effects of divalproex sodium seem to be dose related and significantly less when plasma levels are under 125 µg/mL (Bowden et al. 1994). Gastric upset/diarrhea can be minimized with slow increases in dose and dividing the dose if necessary. Weight gain, fatigue, and sedation may also occur as well as transient loss of hair. The latter side effect can sometimes be controlled with selenium and zinc supplementation (Schmidt 1984).

## Opioid Antagonists

The opioid antagonists were first used in subjects with mental retardation and/or autism who engaged in repetitive SIBs such as head banging and self-biting, based on models of addictive behavior and opioid hyperfunction. Open-label reports described variable responses to these agents, but a recent double-blind placebo-controlled trial did not demonstrate efficacy (Willemsen-Swinkels et al. 1995). A single open-label naltrexone treatment of patients engaging in impulsive SIB has been reported in the literature (Roth et al. 1996). Seven patients, all engaging in at least two episodes of impulsive SIB during the previous month, were treated with 50 mg/day for an average of 10.7 weeks. Patients were selected who reported analgesia during impulsive SIB followed by emotional relief. Four of the subjects had personality disorder diagnoses, two were primarily depressed, and the seventh was diagnosed with schizoaffective disorder. Six of the subjects reported a childhood history of severe sexual abuse. Six of the seven patients had the naltrexone added to an ongoing medication regimen. The authors reported that three of the subjects did not engage in impulsive SIB while receiving naltrexone. Of the four who did, all experienced pain rather than analgesia during impulsive SIB, and dysphoria reduction was decreased. Eventually, in six patients impulsive SIB ceased and the seventh had two episodes in 12 weeks as opposed to at least weekly episodes before treatment (Roth et al. 1996). Theoretically, eliminating the soothing qualities of impulsive SIB without teaching the patient other means of affect regulation could escalate other impulsive self-endangering behaviors such as substance abuse, gambling, promiscuous sexual activity, or actual suicide attempts, yet this has not been reported. Placebo response in subjects with personality disorder can be high, but the dramatic results of this open-label study suggest controlled trials of opioid antagonists in impulsive SIB subjects are indicated.

### β-*Adrenergic Antagonists (β-Blockers)*

β-Blockers have been used to treat aggression in a large variety of patient populations including those with traumatic brain injury, attention deficit disorder, schizophrenia, mental retardation, and posttraumatic stress disorder (for review see Haspel 1995). None of the studies was blinded or placebo controlled, but because an impressive number reported decreases in aggression this medication class is briefly discussed. β-Blockers, by decreasing noradrenergic activity, may work by decreasing arousal and response to environmental stimuli. In addition, the blocking of noradrenergic projections to the cortex may increase serotonergic function (Leonard 1993).

Of interest is that both hydrophobic and hydrophilic (relating to central nervous system penetration) agents have been reported to be effective, in addition to both complete antagonists (such as propranolol) and partial agonists (such as pindolol). The latter may result in better resting sympathetic tone and may also produce results within 2 weeks (Greendyke and Kanter 1986) as opposed to propranolol, which may take 4–6 weeks (Kolb et al. 1984; Mattes 1986; Ratey et al. 1986). Many of these open-label trials suggested that β-blockers may decrease impulsive aggression. It should be noted that none of these studies assessed impulsive SIB. In various studies propranolol was given at doses of up to 960 mg/day and pindolol was given at doses of up to 60 mg/day. Pindolol may work via an additional mechanism of serotonin-1A autoreceptor antagonism that serves to increase serotonergic functioning. A significant confounding factor is that many of the subjects in these studies were receiving neuroleptic agents: β-blockers not only can increase neuroleptic levels and by this mechanism possibly decrease aggression but also can antagonize noradrenergic β-receptors and thereby increase the firing rate of dopaminergic neurons and ameliorate aggressive symptoms through the mechanism of akisthisia reduction (Lipinski et al. 1988).

High doses of β-blockers, particularly propranolol, have been used in open-label studies to decrease dissociative symptoms and switch between "alters" in dissociative identity disorder (Braun 1984). Presumably by decreasing dissociation and the attending numbness that may lead to impulsive SIB, β-blockers may decrease this behavior in such patients.

## Neuroleptics

Neuroleptics have not been specifically studied as a treatment for impulsive SIB. The general effects of neuroleptics have been studied in subjects with personality disorder, but these studies have had mixed findings. In one study, individuals meeting DSM-III criteria for BPD, schizotypal personality disorder, or both were treated with thiothixene at an average daily dose of 8.7 mg/day (Goldberg et al. 1986). Additionally, inclusion criteria included the presence of at least one psychotic symptom. Drug–placebo differences were found in a wide range of symptoms, but were found primarily in psychosis/paranoia-type measures. Impulsive SIB was not measured. The appropriate correction for multiple comparisons was not made, and no improvement was found when validated scales were used. The authors concluded that, secondary to high side effects, minimal efficacy, and risks of tardive dyskinesia, only those patients with personality disorder who have marked psychotic symptoms should be considered for treatment with thiothixene (Goldberg et al. 1986).

Another study compared the efficacy of haloperidol, amitriptyline, and placebo in a 5-week double-blind study of acutely decompensated inpatients with BPD (Soloff et al. 1986b, 1989). The authors were struck by findings similar to earlier studies: medication effects were nonspecific and the apparent improvements occurred over a wide range of symptoms including depression, anxiety, hostility, paranoid ideation, and psychoticism. Haloperidol was poorly tolerated secondary to side effects. In the final analysis, haloperidol was not shown to be an effective treatment. No measures of impulsive SIB were obtained.

A double-blind crossover study comparing trifluoperazine, tranylcypromine, carbamazepine, alprazolam, and placebo in inpatients with BPD has been reported (Cowdry and Gardner 1988). Each medication trial lasted 6 weeks. A high dropout rate occurred for each trial, so analyses were performed on all patients staying in treatment for 3 weeks or longer. Only about seven patients in each of the five treatment groups completed the proposed 6 weeks of medication. No improvement was seen in the trifluoperazine phase on any patient- or physician-rated scales. The authors felt trifluoperizine to be ineffective. In a case report, the "chronic and severe self-mutilating behavior" of a woman with BPD dramatically decreased with clozaril treatment of 300 mg/day after she failed to respond to several trials of psychotropic medications and behavioral interventions (Chengappa et al. 1995). There has been little experience with use of atypical antipsychotic agents for impulsive SIB.

In summary, a few studies have demonstrated some decrease in hostility and aggression in subjects with personality disorder who are treated with neuroleptics. No study using neuroleptics has assessed the utility of these medications for impulsive SIB. Neuroleptics are poorly tolerated secondary to prominence of side effects and carry the risk of causing tardive dyskinesia. There are no data at all regarding maintenance treatment. Atypical neuroleptics could hold promise but have not been investigated in impulsive SIB.

## Benzodiazepines

Benzodiazepines have not been investigated for treatment of impulsive SIB, but one controlled study—a crossover study by Cowdry and Gardner (1988)—assessed alprazolam in subjects with BPD. In a separate report to emphasize a cautionary note, the authors enumerated that 7 of 12 patients receiving an average dose of 4.7 mg/day had episodes of serious behavioral dyscontrol and suicidality as compared with only one patient having such events while receiving placebo (D. L. Gardner and Cowdry 1986). Statistically, patients receiving alprazolam did significantly worse than those receiving placebo. This controlled study demonstrates the potentially disinhibiting or pro-aggression/pro-suicide effects of alprazolam. Numerous other reports exist of disinhibition with other benzodiazepines and in different psychiatric disorders (Gardos et al. 1968; Hall and Jaffe 1972; Ryan et al. 1968).

Benzodiazepines also have a significant potential for addiction and their use should be avoided in individuals with a history of drug and/or alcohol abuse or dependence. In BPD, prevalence of substance abuse has been found to be approximately 35%, predominantly alcohol abuse (Dulit et al. 1990). Benzodiazepines are not absolutely contraindicated but should be used with caution. Some patients, particularly those who engage in impulsive SIB secondary to extreme anxiety, may benefit from longer-acting benzodiazepines such as clonazepam. Alone, benzodiazepines are not lethal in overdose but become so when combined with other central nervous system depressants such as alcohol.

## Monoamine Oxidase Inhibitors

The MAOIs have demonstrated some efficacy in treatment of patients with hysteroid, or rejection-sensitive, dysphoria, which has significant diagnostic overlap with what today we term BPD. Many patients with BPD will engage in impulsive SIB as a means of modulating the overwhelming emotional response they may have to a real or perceived rejection. Decreasing sensitivity to rejection could therefore theoretically decrease impulsive SIB in response to such a situation. In a pilot study comparing five patients who continued to receive phenelzine with six patients who were discontinued, the former group was considered to be significantly improved with regard to depression, anxiety, demanding attitude, dependency, emotional overactivity, and tendency to blame others (Liebowitz and Klein 1979, 1981). This small sample precluded meaningful statistical analysis on many measures and did not assess for impulsive SIB. Additionally, of the five patients who received the MAOI, two experienced a "highly erratic and unsuccessful treatment response."

The crossover study by Cowdry and Gardner (1988) assessed the efficacy of the MAOI tranylcypromine in 12 patients with BPD. This was the only medication among three others for which both physician and patient ratings showed significant improvement compared with those for placebo. Patients receiving this MAOI showed decreased anxiety and rage. Caveats of brief trial length, too small a sample size, possible medication carryover effects, and inadequate correction for multiple comparisons apply. However, tranylcypramine was found to be ineffective in decreasing behavioral dyscontrol compared with carbamazepine in this trial. A double-blind placebo-controlled trial of phenelzine in 34 acute inpatients with BPD failed to show efficacy for this medication (Soloff et al. 1993). Trial length and medication dose, however, may have been insufficient. Both authors discussed the high rate of sleep disturbances, problems with orthostatic hypertension, and the hazards of hypertensive crises that necessitate adherence to dietary restrictions. These factors, in addition to the dangers of overdose and issues of dietary compliance that necessitate avoidance of various illicit and prescription drugs and foods, present the clinician with significant dilemmas in the prescription of MAOIs to impulsive patients.

## Tricyclic Antidepressants

The TCAs have not been studied specifically as a treatment for impulsive SIB. However, TCAs may increase psychologic experiences associated with this disorder. Some of the earliest reports come from the treatment of emotionally unstable patients with character disorder with imipramine, which resulted in increased anger (Klein 1968). In a double-blind placebo-controlled study of amitriptyline in patients with BPD, the authors had the "distinct impression" that many patients receiving amitriptyline became progressively worse, as manifest by increased anxiety, hostility, agitation, dissociative experiences, and behavioral impulsivity (Soloff et al. 1986a). Symptom severity appeared proportional to plasma level of amitriptyline and trial duration. In a later paper reporting final outcome analyses, 57.7%

of patients worsened on hostile depression measures and 64% of patients worsened on schizotypal factors while receiving amitriptyline (Soloff et al. 1989). In a preliminary report of a double-blind placebo-controlled cross-over trial of lithium and desipramine in patients with BPD, desipramine was found to increase patient irritability, anger, and suicidal symptoms (Links et al. 1990). The pro-aggressive/pro-impulsive effects of the TCAs may relate to inhibition of norepinephrine reuptake. The noradrenergic-serotonergic reuptake inhibitors may also theoretically increase these problematic behaviors secondary to increasing noradrenergic activity, although no reports have as yet documented such an occurrence.

In summary, TCAs have met with little success and may actually be detrimental in the treatment of impulsive patients and increase the likelihood of impulsive SIB. Additional problems associated with TCAs in general are uncomfortable side effects, weight gain, and high lethality in overdose (a particular liability in BPD and other impulsive patient groups who make frequent suicidal gestures and/or true attempts).

## Summary and Conclusions

Impulsive SIB occurs in a rather wide variety of diagnoses, including personality disorders (primarily borderline and antisocial), dissociative disorders, depressive disorders, and eating disorders. Impulsive SIB may also be associated with a variety of psychologic experiences such as dissociation, self-hate, shame, and anger. The motivations for these behaviors most frequently include attempts at affect regulation or self-punishment. Behavioral correlates include heightened impulsivity, outward-directed aggression, and other forms of self-directed aggression such as suicide attempts.

Studies of the neurobiology of impulsive SIB are difficult to conduct secondary to the various heterogeneous elements in phenomenologic and diagnostic classifications and other inherent methodologic difficulties as listed in Table 6–1. A few studies provide rather preliminary indications that serotonergic pathways and endogenous opiates may be involved in this behavior. Other measures associated with impulsive SIB, such as impulsive aggression or suicide attempts, have been more clearly related to decreased serotonergic functioning.

The most effective treatment of impulsive SIB involves a combination of psychotherapy and psychopharmacology. The latter also requires a stable therapeutic alliance, given the tendency of those patients who engage in impulsive SIB to have unstable moods, poor coping skills, interpersonal difficulties, and strong transference reactions. These features may result from the experience of childhood trauma, including sexual and physical abuse, or a generally unempathic or invalidating environment.

No medications have received U.S. Food and Drug Administration approval for the treatment of impulsive SIB, nor have any double-blind placebo-controlled trials of medications been performed. Again, positive medication effects in the prototypic impulsive SIB disorder, BPD, are not limited to those symptoms most closely identified to the medication class (i.e., SSRIs work for more than depression, antipsychotic agents may help more than psychotic symptoms). SSRIs, however, have been clearly demonstrated to decrease impulsive-aggressive behaviors and in open-label trials have also been found to decrease impulsive SIB. These medications are well tolerated and are usually a good first choice in pharmacologic treatment of the patient engaging in impulsive SIB. Mood stabilizers, particularly divalproex sodium, may be effective for decreasing impulsive-aggressive behaviors and are also relatively safe medications. Other patients may benefit from particular targeting of symptoms that may be specifically associated with their SIBs. Examples include the use of β-blockers for dissociation, opioid antagonists for impulsive SIB associated with analgesia, MAOIs for rejection sensitivity, and antipsychotic agents for experiences of disintegration, paranoia, and attendant overwhelming anxiety. Little data are available on long-term efficacy of pharmacologic treatments, but there are some indications that treatment response in certain situations may be relatively short lived.

Effective pharmacologic treatment of impulsive SIB involves an ongoing collaborative and integrated treatment approach among the patient, psychiatrist, and therapist if the treatment is "split." Controlled studies are required to better delineate the efficacy of various medications and their particular indications. Despite the high attendant morbidity and mortality associated with impulsive SIB, this area remains remarkably understudied from a pharmacologic standpoint.

## References

American Psychiatric Association: Diagnostic and Statistical Manual of Mental Disorders, 3rd Edition Revised. Washington, DC, American Psychiatric Association, 1987

American Psychiatric Association: Diagnostic and Statistical Manual of Mental Disorders, 4th Edition. Washington, DC, American Psychiatric Association, 1994

Amir S, Brown ZW, Amil A: The role of endorphins in stress: evidence and speculations. Neurosci Behav Rev 4:77–86, 1980

Arango V, Ernsberger P, Marzuk PM, et al: Autoradiographic demonstration of increased serotonin 5-HT2 and beta-adrenergic receptor binding sites in the brains of suicide victims. Arch Gen Psychiatry 47:1038–1047, 1990

Arora RC, Meltzer MY: Serotonin measures in the brains of suicide victims: 5HT2 binding sites in the frontal cortex of suicide victims and control subjects. Am J Psychiatry 146:730–736, 1989

Asberg M, Traskman L, Thoren P: 5-HIAA in the cerebrospinal fluid: a biochemical suicide predictor? Arch Gen Psychiatry 33:1193–1197, 1976

Aston-Jones G, Bloom FE: Norepinephrine-containing locus coeruleus neurons in behaving rats exhibit pronounced responses to non-noxious environmental stimuli. J Neurosci 1:887–890, 1981

Bach-Y-Rita G, Lion JR, Climent CE, et al: Episodic dyscontrol: a study of 130 violent patients. Am J Psychiatry 127:49–54, 1971

Balfour JA, Bryson HM: Valproic acid: a review of its pharmacology and therapeutic potential in indications other than epilepsy. CNS Drugs 2:144–173, 1994

Barrett ES, Kent TA, Byrant SG, et al: A controlled trial of phenytoin in impulsive aggression. J Clin Psychopharmacol 11:388–389, 1992

Barrett RP, Feinstein C, Hole WT: Effects of naloxone and naltrexone on self-injury: a double-blind, placebo-controlled analysis. Am J Ment Retard 93:644–651, 1989

Barron JL, Sandman CA: Paradoxical excitement to sedative-hypnotics in mentally retarded clients. Am J Ment Defic 90:124–129, 1985

Bernstein GA, Hughes JR, Mitchell JE, et al: Effects of narcotic antagonists on self-injurious behavior: a single case study. J Am Acad Child Adolesc Psychiatry 26:886–889, 1987

Biegon A, Grinspoon A, Blumenfeld B, et al: Increased serotonin 5-HT2 receptor binding on blood platelets of suicidal men. Psychopharmacology (Berl) 100:165–167, 1990

Blumer D, Heibronn M, Himmelhoch J: Indications for carbamazepine in mental illness: atypical psychiatric disorder or temporal lobe syndrome? Compr Psychiatry 29:108–122, 1988

Bowden CL, Brugger AM, Swann AC: Efficacy of divalproex vs lithium and placebo in the treatment of mania. JAMA 271:918–924, 1994

Braun BG: Towards a theory of multiple personality and other dissociative phenomena. Psychiatr Clin North Am 7:171–193, 1984

Brown CS, Kent TA, Bryant SG, et al: Blood platelet uptake of serotonin in episodic aggression. Psychiatry Res 27:5–12, 1989

Brown GL, Ballenger JC, Goyer PF, et al: Aggression in humans correlates with cerebrospinal fluid metabolites. Psychiatry Res 1:131–139, 1979

Brown GL, Ebert MH, Goyer PF, et al: Aggression, suicide, and serotonin: relationships to CSF amine metabolites. Am J Psychiatry 139:741–746, 1982

Brunner HG, Nelen MR, van Zandvoort P, et al: X-linked borderline mental retardation with prominent behavioral disturbance: phenotype, genetic localization, and evidence for disturbed monoamine metabolism. Am J Hum Genet 52:1032–1039, 1993

Cases O, Seif I, Grimsby J, et al: Aggressive behavior and altered amounts of brain serotonin and norepinephrine in mice lacking MAOA. Science 268:1763–1776, 1995

Cates DS, Houston BK, Vavak CR, Crawford MH et al: Heritability of hostility-related emotions, attitudes, and behaviors. J Behav Med 16:237–256, 1993

Chen D, Rainnie DG, Greene RW, et al: Abnormal fear response and aggressive behavior in mutant mice deficient for $\alpha$-calcium-calmodulin kinase II. Science 266:291–294, 1994

Chengappa RKN, Baker RW, Sirri C: The successful use of clazapine in ameliorating severe self mutilation in a patient with borderline personality disorder. J Personal Disord 9:76–82, 1995

Clarkin J, Widiger T, Frances A: A prototypic typology and the borderline personality disorder. J Abnorm Psychol 92:263–275, 1983

Coccaro EF, Kavoussi RJ: Fluoxetine and impulsive-aggressive behavior in personality-disordered subjects. Arch Gen Psychiatry 54:1081–1088, 1997

Coccaro EF, Siever LJ, Klar HM, et al: Serotonergic studies in patients with affective and personality disorders. Arch Gen Psychiatry 47:587–599, 1989

Coccaro EF, Astill JL, Herbert JA: Fluoxetine treatment of impulsive aggression in refractory borderline patients. J Clin Pharmacol 10:373–375, 1990a

Coccaro EF, Gabriel S, Siever LJ: Buspirone challenge: Preliminary evidence for a role for central 5-HT$_{1A}$ receptor function in impulsive-aggressive behavior in humans. Psychopharmacol Bull 26:393–405, 1990b

Coccaro EF, Lawrence T, Trestman R, et al: Growth hormone responses to intravenous clonidine challenge correlate with behavioral irritability in psychiatric patients and healthy volunteers. Psychiatry Res 39:129–139, 1991

Coccaro EF, Bergeman CS, McClearn GE: Heritability of irritable impulsiveness: a study of twins reared together and apart. Psychiatry Res 48:229–242, 1993

Coccaro EF, Kavoussi RJ, Hauger RL: Physiological responses to d-fenfluramine and ipsapirone challenge correlate with indices of aggression in males with personality disorder. Int Clin Psychopharmacol 10:177–179, 1995

Coccaro EF, Kavoussi RJ, Sheline YI, et al: Impulsive aggression in personality disorder correlates with tritiated paroxetine binding in the platelet. Arch Gen Psychiatry 53:531–536, 1996

Coccaro EF, Kavoussi RJ, Cooper TB, et al: Central serotonin activity and aggression: inverse relationship with prolactin response to d-fenfluramine, but not CSF 5-HIAA concentration, in human subjects. Am J Psychiatry 154:1430–1435, 1997a

Coccaro EF, Kavoussi RJ, Sheline YI, et al: Impulsive aggression in personality disorder: correlates with [125]I-LSD binding in the platelet. Neuropsychopharmacology 6:211–216, 1997b

Coid J, Allolio B, Rees LH: Raised plasma metenkephalin in patients who habitually mutilate themselves. Lancet 2:545–546, 1983

Cornelius JR, Soloff PH, Perel JM, et al: Fluoxetine trial in borderline personality disorder. Psychopharmacol Bull 26:151–154, 1990

Cowdry RW, Gardner DL: Pharmacotherapy of borderline personality disorder: alprazolam, carbamazepine, trifluoperazine, and tranylcypromine. Arch Gen Psychiatry 45:111–119, 1988

Davidson PW, Kleene BM, Carroll M, et al: Effect of naloxone on self-injurious behavior: a case study. Appl Res Ment Retard 4:1–4, 1983

Deltito JA: The effect of valproate on bipolar spectrum tempermental disorders. J Clin Psychiatry 54:300–304, 1993

Dulit RA, Fyer MR, Haas GL: Substance use in borderline personality disorder. Am J Psychiatry 147:1002–1007, 1990

Eichelman B, Barchas J: Facilitated shock-induced aggression following antidepressant medication in the rat. 3:601–604, 1975

Favazza AR, Conterio K: Female habitual self-mutilators. Acta Psychiatr Scand 79:283–289, 1989

Gardner AR, Gardner AJ: Self-mutilation, obsessionality, and narcissism. Br J Psychiatry 127:127–132, 1975

Gardner DL, Cowdry RW: Alprazolam-induced dyscontrol in borderline personality disorder. Am J Psychiatry 42:98–100, 1985

Gardner DL, Cowdry RW: Development of melancholia during carbamazepine treatment in borderline personality disorder. J Clin Psychopharmacol 6:236–239, 1986

Gardner DL, Lucas PB, Cowdry RW: CSF metabolites in borderline personality disorder compared with normal controls. Biol Psychiatry 28:247–254, 1990

Gardos G, DiMasio A, Salzman C: Differential actions of chlorodiazepoxide and oxazepam on hostility. Arch Gen Psychiatry 18:757–760, 1968

Giakas WJ, Seibyl JP, Mazure CM: Valproate in the treatment of temper outbursts (letter). J Clin Psychiatry 51:525, 1990

Goldberg SC, Schulz SC, Schulz PM, et al: Borderline and schizotypal personality disorders treated with low-dose thiothixene vs placebo. Arch Gen Psychiatry 43:680–686, 1986

Goyer PF, Andreason PJ, Semple WE, et al: Positron-emission tomography and personality disorders. Neuropsychopharmacology 10:21–28, 1994

Greendyke RM, Kanter DM: Therapeutic effects of pindolol on behavioral disturbances associated with organic brain disease: a double-blind study. J Clin Psychiatry 47:423–426, 1986

Grunebaum HV, Klerman GL: Wrist slashing. Am J Psychiatry 124:527–534, 1967

Hall RC, Jaffe JR: Aberrant response to diazepam: a new syndrome. Am J Psychiatry 129:738–742, 1972

Hasan MY, Sewell RDE, Nicholls PJ: Does the anticonvulsant agent sodium valproate display behaviorally selective anti-offensive activity? Journal of Pharmacy and Pharmacology 42(suppl):185, 1990

Haspel T: Beta-blockers and the treatment of aggression. Harv Rev Psychiatry 2:274–281, 1995

Herman BH: A possible role of proopiomelanocortin peptides in self-injurious behavior. Prog Neuropsychopharmacol Biol Psychiatry 14:109–139, 1990

Herman BH, Hammock MK, Arthur-Smith A, et al: Naltrexone decreases self-injurious behavior. Ann Neurol 22:550qP552, 1987

Hilakivi-Clarke LA, Corduban TD, Tairi T, et al: Alterations in brain monoamines and GABA$_A$ receptors in transgenic mice over-expressing TGFα. Pharmacol Biochem Behav 40:593–600, 1995

Hollander E, Grossman R, Stein D et al: Borderline personality disorder and impulsive-aggression: the role for divalproex sodium treatment. Psychiatr Ann 26(suppl):464–469, 1996

Jacobsen FM: Low-dose valproate: a new treatment for cyclothymia, mild rapid cycling disorders, and premenstrual syndrome. J Clin Psychiatry 54:229–234, 1993

Kavoussi RJ, Liu J, Coccaro EF: An open trial of sertraline in personality disordered patients with impulsive aggression. J Clin Psychiatry 55:137–141, 1994

Keck PE, McElroy SL, Friedman LM: Valproate and carbamazepine in the treatment of panic and posttraumatic stress disorders, withdrawal states, and behavioral dyscontrol syndromes. J Clin Psychopharmacol 12(suppl):36–41, 1992

Klein DF: Psychiatric diagnosis and topology of clinical drug effects. Psychopharmacology 13:359–386, 1968

Koenigsberg HW: A comparison of hospitalized and nonhospitalized borderline patients. Am J Psychiatry 139:1292–1297, 1982

Kolb LS, Burris, B, Griffith S: Propranolol and Clonidine in the Treatment of the Chronic Posttraumatic Stress Disorder: Psychological and Biological Sequelae. Washington, DC, American Psychiatric Press, 1984, pp 98–105

Konig M, Zimmer AM, Steiner H, et al: Pain responses, anxiety and aggression in mice deficient in pre-proenkephalin. Nature 383:535–538, 1996

Kravitz HM, Fawcett J: Carbemazepine in the treatment of affective disorders. Med Sci Res 15:1–8, 1987

Leibenluft E, Gardner DL, Cowdry RW: The inner experience of the borderline self-mutilator. J Personal Disord 1:317–324, 1987

Leonard BE: The comparative pharmacology of new antidepressants. J Clin Psychiatry 54(suppl):3–15, 1993

Lesch KP, Mayer S, Disselkamp-Tietze J, et al: 5-HT$_{1A}$ receptor responsivity in unipolar depression: evaluation of ipsapirone-induced ACTH and cortisol secretion in patients and controls. Biol Psychiatry 28:620–628, 1990a

Lesch KP, Mayer S, Disselkamp-Tietze J, et al: Subsensitivity of the 5-hydroxytryptamine 1A (5-HT$_{1A}$) receptor-mediated hypothermic response to ipsapirone in unipolar depression. Life Sci 46:1271–1277, 1990b

Lesch K, Bengel D, Heils A, et al: Association of anxiety-related traits with a polymorphism in the serotonin transporter gene regulatory region. Science 274:1527–1531, 1996

Liebowitz MR, Klein DF: Hysteroid dysphoria. Psychiatr Clin North Am 2:555–575, 1979

Liebowitz MR, Klein DF: Interrelationship of hysteroid dysphoria and borderline personality disorder. Psychiatr Clin North Am 4:67–87, 1981

Links PS, Steiner M, Boiago I, et al: Lithium therapy for borderline patients: preliminary findings. J Clin Psychopharmacol 4:173–181, 1990

Linnoila M, Virkunnen M, Scheinin M, et al: Low cerebrospinal fluid 5-hydroxyindoleacetic acid concentration differentiates impulsive from non-impulsive violent behavior. Life Sci 33:2609–2614, 1983

Lipinski JF, Keck PE, McElroy SL: β-Adrenergic antagonists in psychosis: is improvement due to treatment of neuroleptic-induced akathisia? J Clin Psychopharmacol 8:406–416, 1988

Madden J, Akil H, Patrick R, et al: Stress-induced parallel changes in central opioid levels and pain responsiveness in the rat. Nature 265:358–360, 1977

Maletsky BM: The episodic dyscontrol syndrome. Dis Nerv Syst 34:178–185, 1973

Mann JJ, Malone KM, Diehl DJ, et al: Demonstration in vivo of reduced serotonin responsivity in the brain of untreated depressed patients. Am J Psychiatry 153:174–182, 1996

Markowitz P: Pharmacotherapy of impulsivity, aggression, and related disorders, in Impulsivity and Aggression. Edited by Hollander E, Stein D. New York, John Wiley and Sons, 1995, pp 260–280

Markowitz PJ, Wagner SC: Venlafaxine in the treatment of borderline personality disorder. Psychopharmocol Bull 31:773–777, 1995

Markowitz PJ, Calabrese JR, Schulz SC: Fluoxetine treatment of borderline and schizotypal personality disorder. Am J Psychiatry 148:1064–1067, 1991

Mattes JA: Propranolol for adults with temper outbursts and residual attention deficit disorder. J Clin Psychopharmacol 6:299–302, 1986

Mattes J: Comparative effectiveness of carbamazepine and propranolol for rage outbursts. J Neuropsychiatry Clin Neurosci 2:159–164, 1990

McElroy SL, Keck PE Jr, Pope HG Jr: Sodium valproate: its use in primary psychiatric disorders. J Clin Psychopharmacol 7:16–24, 1987

New AS, Trestman RL, Mitropoulou V, et al: Serotonergic function and self-injurious behavior in personality disorder patients. Psychiatry Res 69:17–26, 1997

New AS, Gelernter J, Yovell Y, et al: Tryptophan hydroxylase genotype is associated with impulsive-aggressive measures: a preliminary study. Am J Med Genet 81:13–17, 1998

Nielsen DA, Goldman D, Virkkunen M, et al: Suicidality and 5-hydroxyindolacetic acid concentration associated with a tryptophan hydroxylase polymorphism. Arch Gen Psychiatry 51:34–38, 1994

Norden NJ: Fluoxetine in borderline personality disorder. Prog Neuropsychopharmacol Biol Psychiatry 13:885–893, 1989

Panksepp J, Herman B, Conner R, et al: The biology of social attachment: opiates alleviate separation distress. Biol Psychiatry 13:607–618, 1978

Pauls AM, Lautenbacher S, Strian F, et al: Assessment of somatosensory indicators of polyneuropathy in patients with eating disorders. Eur Arch Psychiatry Clin Neurosci 241:8–12, 1991

PDR (Physician's Desk Reference), 50th Edition. Montvale, NJ, Medical Economics 1996

Rasmussen K, Strecker RE, Jacobs BL: Single unit response of locus coeruleus in the freely moving cat, I: during naturalistic behaviors and in response to simple and complex stimuli. Brain Res 371:324–334, 1986

Ratey JJ, Mikkelsen EJ, Smith GB, et al: β-Blockers in the severely and profoundly mentally retarded. J Clin Psychopharmacol 6:103–107, 1986

Richardson JS, Zaleski WA: Naloxone and self-mutilation. Biol Psychiatry 18:99–101, 1983

Richardson JS, Zaleski WA: Endogenous opiates and self-mutilation. Am J Psychiatry 143:938–940, 1986

Rifkin A, Quitkin F, Curillo C: Lithium carbonate in emotionally unstable character disorder. Arch Gen Psychiatry 27:519–523, 1972

Ross RR, McKay HB: Self-Mutilation. Lexington, MA, Lexington Books, 1979

Roth AS, Ostroff RB, Hoffman RE: Naltrexone as a treatment for repetitive self-injurious behavior: an open-label trial. J Clin Psychiatry 57:233–237, 1996

Roy A: Self-mutilation. Br J Med Psychol 51:201–203, 1978

Roy A, DeJong J, Linnoila M: Extraversion in pathological gamblers: correlates with indexes of noradrenergic function. Arch Gen Psychiatry 46:679–681, 1989

Rushton JP, Fulker DW, Neale MC, et al: Altruism and aggression: the heritability of individual differences. J Personal Soc Psychol 50:1192–1198, 1986

Russ MJ, Roth SD, Lerman A, et al: Pain perception in self-injurious patients with borderline personality disorder. Biol Psychiatry 32:501–511, 1992

Russ MJ, Shearin EN, Clarkin JF, et al: Subtypes of self-injurious patients with borderline personality disorder. Am J Psychiatry 150:1869–1871, 1993

Russ MJ, Roth SD, Kakuma T, et al: Pain perception in self-injurious borderline patients: naloxone effects. Biol Psychiatry 35:207–209, 1994

Ryan HF, Merrill FB, Scott GE: Increase in suicidal thoughts and tendencies: association with diazepam therapy. JAMA 203:1137–1139, 1968

Sandman CA, Datta PC, Barron J, et al: Naloxone attenuates self-abusive behavior in developmentally disabled clients. Appl Res Ment Retard 4:5–11, 1983

Sandyk R: Naloxone abolishes self-injuring in a mentally retarded child (letter). Ann Neurol 17:520, 1985

Saudou F, Amara DA, Dierich A, et al: Enhanced aggressive behavior in mice lacking 5-$HT_{1B}$ receptor. Science 265:1875–1878, 1994

Schaff MR, Fawcett J, Zajecka JM: Divalproex sodium in the treatment of refractory affective disorders. J Clin Psychiatry 54:380–384, 1993

Schiff HB, Sabin TD, Geller A, et al: Lithium in aggressive behavior. Am J Psychiatry 139:1346–1348, 1982

Schmidt D: Adverse effects of valproate. Epilepsia 25:44–49, 1984

Sheard M, Marini J, Bridges C, et al: The effect of lithium on impulsive-aggressive behavior in man. Am J Psychiatry 133:1409–1413, 1976

Siever LJ, Trestman RL: The serotonin system and aggressive personality disorder. Int Clin Psychopharmacol 8(suppl):33–39, 1993

Simeon D, Stanley B, Frances A, et al: Self-mutilation in personality disorders: psychological and biological correlates. Am J Psychiatry 149:221–226, 1992

Soloff PH, Anselm G, Nathan RS, et al: Paradoxical effects of amitriptyline on borderline patients. Am J Psychiatry 143:1603–1605, 1986a

Soloff PH, George A, Nathan RS, et al: Progress in pharmacotherapy of borderline disorders: a double-blind study of amitriptyline, haloperidol, and placebo. Arch Gen Psychiatry 43:691–697, 1986b

Soloff PH, George A, Nathan RS, et al: Amitriptyline versus haloperidol in borderlines: final outcomes and predictors of response. J Clin Psychopharmacol 9:238–246, 1989

Soloff PH, Cornelius J, George A, et al: Efficacy of phenelzine and haloperidol in borderline personality disorder. Arch Gen Psychiatry 50:377–385, 1993

Stein DJ, Simeon D, Frenkel M, et al: An open label trial of valproate in borderline personality disorder. J Clin Psychiatry 56:506–510, 1995

Steinberg BJ, Trestman R, Mitroupoulou V, et al: Depressive response to physostigmine challenge in borderline personality disorder patients. Neuropsychopharmacology 17:264–273, 1997

Sternbach RA: Pain: A Psychophysiological Analysis. New York, Academic Press, 1968

Stoff DM, Pollock L, Vitello B, et al: Reduction of (3M)-imipramine binding sites on platelets of conduct-disorder children. Neuropsychopharmacology 1:55–62, 1987

Stolk JM, Conner RL, Levine S, et al: Brain norepinephrine metabolism and shock-induced fighting behavior in rats: differential effects of shock and fighting on the neurochemical response to a common footshock stimulus. J Pharmacol Exp Ther 190:193–209, 1974

Teicher MH, Glod C, Cole JO: Emergence of intense suicidal preoccupation during fluoxetine treatment. Am J Psychiatry 147:207–210, 1990

Tellegen A, Lykken DT, Bouchard TJ, et al: Personality similarity in twins reared apart and together. J Personal Soc Psychol 54:1031–1039, 1988

van der Kolk BA, Greenberg MS, Orr SP, et al: Endogenous opioids, stress-induced analgesia, and posttraumatic stress disorder. Psychopharmacol Bull 25:417–421, 1989

Virkkunen M, Nuutila A, Goodwin FK, et al: Cerebrospinal fluid monoamine metabolite levels in male arsonists. Arch Gen Psychiatry 44:241–247, 1987

Widiger TA, Rogers JH: Prevalence and comorbidity of personality disorders. Psychiatr Ann 19:132–136, 1989

Willemsen-Swinkels SH, Buitelaar JK, Nijhof GJ, et al: Failure of naltrexone hydrochloride to reduce self-injurious and autistic behavior in mentally retarded adults. Arch Gen Psychiatry 52:766–773, 1995

Zarate CA Jr, Tohen M, Banov MD, et al: Is clozapine a mood stabilizer? J Clin Psychiatry 56:108–112, 1995

# CHAPTER 7

# Dialectical Behavior Therapy for Impulsive Self-Injurious Behaviors

Andre Ivanoff, Ph.D.
Marsha M. Linehan, Ph.D.
Milton Brown, M.A.

## Introduction

The term *parasuicide* refers to any nonfatal self-injurious behavior (SIB) with clear intent to cause bodily harm or death that results in actual tissue damage, illness, or risk of death (Kreitman 1977). Parasuicide is a heterogeneous category that includes both SIB with lethal intent and SIB without lethal intent. *Self-mutilation* refers to the deliberate infliction of direct physical injury—for example, piercing, scratching, cutting, or burning—to one's own body without intent to die (Winchel and Stanley 1991) and is usually viewed as distinct from other forms of parasuicide such as deliberate overdoses or self-poisoning. Wrist cutting or skin burning, for example, are forms of self-mutilation that, in contrast to suicide attempts, are typically considered more repetitive and pose lower risk of death (Bach-Y-Rita 1974; A.R. Gardner and Gardner 1975; Graff and Mallin 1967; Morgan 1979; Pao 1969; Pattison and Kahan 1983; Ross et al. 1978; Simpson 1976; Walsh 1987; Walsh and Rosen 1988; Widiger and Weissman 1991).

Confusion exists, however, in how parasuicide is categorized. One problem is that most deliberate parasuicide involves ambivalent intent to die (Brown and Linehan 1996; Walsh 1987). Similarly, the correlations among self-mutilation, suicidal behavior, and suicidal ideation also create problems in forming discrete categories. For example, 40% of one sample of self-cutters reported a wish to die at the time of their low lethality mutilation (I.H. Jones et al. 1979), and in two other studies (A.R. Gardner and Gardner 1975; Pattison and Kahan 1983), 41% and 28% of self-mutilators cited suicidal thoughts as associated with their self-mutilating acts (see Linehan 1997a for a review of other classification problems). Among self-mutilating adolescents, 31% made a serious suicide attempt close to the time of their self-mutilation (Walsh 1987). More generally, other studies show that 50%–90% of those who engage in nonsuicidal self-mutilation also engage in suicidal behavior (Favazza and Conterio 1989; Hillbrand et al. 1994; Simeon et al. 1992). In a sample of 61 women with borderline personality disorder (BPD) who had engaged in parasuicide, 43% had engaged in both a suicidal and a nonsuicidal act (mostly cutting or burning) during the past year (Brown and Linehan 1996). Other problems obfuscating parasuicide categories arise from the difficulty of reliably inferring intent. Assessment of intent may be biased by the interviewer's theory of such behavior, by temporality (i.e., when assessment is conducted), or by assumptions that are made about consequences, such as the notion that low-lethality behavior carries no suicidal intent. This chapter describes Dialectical Behavior Therapy (DBT), a model of treatment for parasuicide including self-mutilation, in women with BPD. Special attention is given to treatment procedures recommended for behavioral and cognitive characteristics associated with self-mutilation.

## Self-Mutilation and Borderline Personality Disorder

Parasuicide, including self-mutilation and suicidal behavior, is considered to be a common clinical behavior among individuals who are diagnosed with BPD. The characteristics associated with those who parasuicide and with those meeting criteria for BPD are strikingly similar in the literature on suicidal behavior; BPD is the only diagnosis for which parasuicide is a criterion. BPD is generally characterized by intense negative emotions, including depression, self-hatred, anger, and hopelessness, frequently accompanied by anxiety and psychotic symptoms. Difficulty in regulating emotions and behaviors results in unstable and chaotic interpersonal relationships. Patients with BPD often engage in impulsive behaviors such as self-mutilation, alcohol or drug abuse, eating binges, and suicidal behaviors. A significant health problem particularly among women, BPD affects approximately 11% of all psychiatric outpatients and 19% of inpatients; 70%–77% of these are women (Widiger and Frances 1987).

Up to 80% of inpatients with BPD have self-mutilated at some time in the past, approximately 40% have engaged in "nonserious" suicide attempts (Fyer 1988), and up to 55% have made serious suicide attempts (Fyer 1988; Gunderson 1984). Gunderson (1984) called parasuicide the "behavioral specialty" of the patient with BPD. The rate of suicide among these patients is 5%–10% (Frances et al. 1986), which is similar to rates associated with major affective disorder or schizophrenia, the diagnoses with highest suicide rates, and double that when examining only those with a history of previous parasuicide (Stone et al. 1987).

Most parasuicidal acts among patients with BPD lack definite lethal intent and most involve multiple and ambivalent intentions (Brown and Linehan 1996). In a sample of 61 patients with BPD and at least two previous episodes of parasuicide admitted to the University of Washington Behavior Therapy Research Clinic, 30 of the acts were suicide attempts, whereas 31 had no lethal intent associated with them. In the past year, 26 of the 61 patients had both a suicide attempt and nonsuicidal parasuicide, mostly cutting/burning, and 35 of 61 had either a suicide attempt or nonsuicidal parasuicide (Brown and Linehan 1996). In four other studies, 17%–50% of individuals who parasuicided reported a moderate intent to die. In one sample of women meeting criteria for BPD, most mutilation by cutting or burning involved little suicide intent or medical risk when compared with other methods of parasuicide (Brown and Linehan 1996).

When developing an effective model for treating self-mutilation, it is useful to view self-mutilating behavior as a function of limited problem-solving abilities and emotional dysregulation. Parasuicidal individuals lack skillful coping ability in general (see Linehan 1993a and 1993b for review), and dysfunctional problem-solving significantly predicts subsequent parasuicide among parasuicidal borderline women (Kehrer and Linehan 1996). Self-mutilation and other forms of parasuicide may function as problem-solving behaviors in several ways. Several investigators (e.g., Maris 1981; Linehan 1993a, 1993b; Shneidman 1987) have suggested that parasuicide, including both self-mutilation and suicide attempts, may actually help some individuals cope with life problems that cause intense suffering by reducing the emotional pain or cognition linked to the suffering. Parasuicide may also function as problem solving by influencing others in ways that alleviate difficult circumstances or demands or elicit assistance or support (Favazza 1989). Particularly true of behavior such as self-mutilation and suicide threats, some individuals acknowledge engaging in these behaviors to influence others (Leibenluft et al. 1987). In this way, parasuicide may also indirectly serve to reduce painful emotions through interpersonal problem solving. The communication of emotional pain to others may result in validation of that pain, and demonstration of the severity of problems may elicit help or maintain a valued relationship (Linehan 1981; Wagner and Linehan 1997). Finally, suicidal behaviors are one of the most effective means of admission to psychiatric hospitals.

Viewed pejoratively, such acts are seen as manipulative communication (Gunderson 1984). Individuals who engage in these behaviors have limited help-seeking skills (Ivanoff et al. 1992; Linehan et al. 1987; Schotte and Clum 1987), and these communications are often reinforced when the environment becomes more responsive after parasuicide. In this way, extreme behaviors such as self-mutilation and other forms of parasuicide can easily become primary means of problem solving.

## Emotional Dysregulation and Self-Mutilation

Individuals who self-mutilate and parasuicide may also experience persistent and acute emotional dysregulation. BPD is widely characterized by severe emotional lability and reactivity (Linehan 1993a, 1993b). Self-mutilating individuals are generally assessed as more angry and more verbally and physically aggressive than nonparasuicidal individuals with psychiatric illness (Hillbrand et al. 1994; Roy 1978; Simeon et al. 1992). Self-mutilators also attribute their own behavior to uncontrolled anger (Roy 1978).

Emotional dysregulation may be functionally viewed as the result of emotional vulnerability (which includes both a predisposition to intense and long-lasting emotional reactions and a low threshold for emotional activation) combined with a lack of skillful ways to regulate distressing emotions. Emotional dysregulation occupies a central role in self-mutilation. Negative emotions appear to play a role in self-mutilation through the process of negative reinforcement—that is, the reduction of negative emotions after mutilation (emotional catharsis in psychodynamic terms [D.L. Gardner and Cowdry 1985]). Patients typically report experiencing intolerable anxiety and tension, often accompanied by depersonalization or emptiness, that is usually relieved after self-mutilation (Favazza 1989; Favazza and Conterio 1989; A.R. Gardner and Gardner 1975; A. Jones 1986; Kemperman et al. 1997; Rosenthal et al. 1972; Simeon et al. 1992; Simpson 1976; Wilkinson and Coid 1991).

Interviews with self-mutilating patients who experienced childhood incest and adult rape suggest that depersonalization occurs when tension associated with posttraumatic stress from sexual abuse becomes intolerable. Self-mutilation reportedly alleviates these negative states (Greenspan and Samuel 1989; Shapiro 1987). Women with BPD report that parasuicid-al behavior may reduce dissociation in response to painful emotions, thus enabling them to avoid numbness and disconnection from reality (Wagner and Linehan 1997). Other investigators report that patterns of repeated, low-lethality self-mutilation are associated with poor tolerance of anxiety and anger (D.L. Gardner and Cowdry 1985; Pattison and Kahan 1983). An analogue study employing psychophysiologic measurement strongly suggests that self-mutilation is associated with a quick reduction of negative emotional arousal (Haines et al. 1996). Taken together, these data suggest that self-mutilation may be strengthened and maintained because of the physiologic and emotional reinforcement of this effective, albeit maladaptive, coping strategy.

Shame appears to be a critically important emotion in self-mutilation. Clinical observation supports the relationship between self-mutilation and negative attitude toward the self. Early theorists were first to suggest that anger toward the self leads to nonsuicidal self-mutilation (Freud 1949; Liebowitz 1987). Patients who chronically self-mutilate or those who meet criteria for BPD often view themselves as evil and deserving punishment and frequently experience shame, guilt, and self-hatred (Anderson 1981; Leibenluft et al. 1987; Linehan 1993a, 1993b; Shapiro 1987; Walsh and Rosen 1988). The association of shame and self-mutilation may also explain the relationship of self-mutilation to sexual abuse. Self-mutilation, suicide attempts, and diagnosis of BPD correlate strongly and uniquely with childhood sexual abuse. Self-mutilation can follow adult rape (Greenspan and Samuel 1989) and is described as the result of self-hatred and shame among women with histories of sexual abuse who report blaming themselves for their own pain and for that of their family members (Shapiro 1987). Similarly, adolescents who self-mutilated close to the time of reporting sexual abuse led Anderson (1981) to conclude that sexual abuse results in self-mutilation in part because of self-blame and shame.

Several prospective studies have suggested a link between shame and self-mutilation. Self-derogation predicted parasuicide in the earliest study (Kaplan and Pokorny 1969), whereas more recently, current level of shame (but not other emotions) predicted increases in urges to self-harm when talking about recent personal parasuicide (Brown and Linehan 1996), which suggests that current shame is a vulnerability to urges to harm oneself. High levels of shame but not other emotions before starting therapy also substantially increased the odds that a patient self-mutilated within the first 4 months of therapy. Shame continued to predict parasuicide even when the total number of parasuicide acts during the past year and other negative emotions were controlled (Brown et al. 1997).

## Dialectical Behavior Therapy

Dialectical behavior therapy (Linehan 1993a, 1993b) is a treatment that addresses the factors related to self-mutilation and has been found effective at reducing the incidence and frequency of all forms of parasuicide in women diagnosed with BPD. Designated as an empirically validated treatment by the American Psychological Association (1993), it is the first psychotherapy for the behaviors associated with BPD supported by randomized clinical trials. DBT originally was developed by Linehan and colleagues at the University of Washington as a treatment for chronically parasuicidal women (Linehan 1993a, 1993b). Over time, it became clear that most of these women also met criteria for BPD, and the treatment evolved accordingly.

Standard DBT is a 1-year outpatient treatment based on social learning theory, employing primarily behavioral and cognitive-behavioral methods. Patients participate simultaneously in both weekly individual psychotherapy and in skills training groups that teach adaptive coping skills in the four primary problem areas attributed to BPD: 1) emotion regulation, 2) distress tolerance, 3) interpersonal effectiveness, and 4) reduction of confusion about identity and maladaptive cognition ("mindfulness") (Linehan 1993a, 1993b). Individual treatment addresses specific maladaptive behaviors while strengthening and generalizing skills. Corollary treatment components include patient telephone consultation, treatment team supervision, and ongoing consultation with the therapist. Both the individual psychotherapy and the skills training group are necessary components in DBT. The individual psychotherapy components of DBT provide the relationship and context in which patients use new skills to gain control over self-harm and suicidal behaviors. Many inpatient day-treatment programs and outpatient practices implement DBT by starting with skills training groups or on an individual basis. Skills training alone, however, should not be confused with comprehensive DBT, as data below indicate.

### Empirical Support

In the first DBT clinical trial (Linehan et al. 1991), 47 chronically parasuicidal women who met criteria for BPD were randomly assigned to either 12 months of DBT or a community treatment as usual. Assessments occurred every 4 months during treatment and at 12-month follow-up. Results showed that DBT clients were less likely to engage in any form of parasuicide or to drop out of therapy than therapy-as-usual clients. The DBT group also spent less time in psychiatric hospitals, was better adjusted interpersonally, was less angry, and maintained significantly higher Global Assessment Scale scores (Endicott et al. 1976) than did the therapy-as-usual subjects (Linehan 1993a). Reanalysis of the data (Linehan and Heard 1993) confirmed that the overall superiority of DBT was not accounted for by the fact that DBT patients had greater access to psychotherapy and to telephone consultation than did therapy-as-usual patients. The mean number of self-mutilation acts was somewhat lower among DBT patients, but the difference was not significant. The effectiveness of skills training alone was also examined, minus individual DBT therapy or with skills coaching between sessions. Skills training alone, without coaching, was not effective as an additive treatment to ongoing DBT individual psychotherapy. Individuals in this study (Linehan and Heard 1993) essentially did no better (or worse) than those in the therapy-as-usual condition in the above described trial (Linehan 1993a).

The second randomized clinical trial and single largest application to date involved substance-abusing women with BPD (Linehan MM, Dimeff LA: "Extension of Standard Dialectical Behavior Therapy to Treatment of Substance Abusers with Borderline Personality Disorder," unpublished manual, 1996). Preliminary outcome data indicate that individuals in the DBT condition decreased drug use more than therapy-as-usual subjects and stayed in treatment longer. At follow-up, the former groups had made significantly greater gains in global and social adjustment than the latter.

Several studies evaluating DBT in suicidal BPD patients have been completed or are currently in progress at sites in the United States and in Europe. Two randomized controlled trials and two studies with parallel comparisons (Barley et al. 1993; Miller et al. 1997) found DBT to be more effective than therapy-as-usual at changing patterns of behavior associated with BPD. Since its inception, DBT has been adapted to various client populations and settings. Telch (1997) developed, adapted, and tested DBT skills training for use with obese women with binge-eating disorder. Other adaptations that show excellent promise, albeit on the basis of uncontrolled data, include adaptation for inpatient psychiatric settings (Swenson et al., in press), DBT for inner-city suicidal adolescents (Miller et al. 1997), day treatment applications (Swenson et al. [in press]), forensic psychiatric settings (including adaptations for both borderline and antisocial personality disorder patients) (Ball E, McCann RA, Ivanoff A, et al.: "DBT in an Inpatient Forensic Setting: Preliminary Outcomes," unpublished manuscript, 1996), and emergency psychiatric settings (McKeon R: "DBT in an Emergency Psychiatric Setting," unpublished manuscript, 1996).

## Biosocial Theory and Procedures

Its dialectical philosophy of treatment, biosocial theory, and treatment stages and targets distinguish DBT from other cognitive-behavioral treatments for BPD. Dialectics function as a world view, a theory of disorder, a model for persuasive dialogue, and as a frame for the interrelationships between individuals or among behaviors, events, and cognition. Furthermore, effective treatment strategies emerge from this basic philosophic stance of dialectics. The theory used to explain BPD is based in a dialectical philosophy that combines both stress-diathesis and learning models of psychopathology as the framework for synthesizing biologic and environmental approaches to the etiology and maintenance of BPD. Dialectical philosophy emphasizes interconnectedness and wholeness; all things are seen as inherently heterogeneous and composed of opposing forces that synthesize to produce change and facilitate the construction of truth over time. Change is therefore viewed as a fundamental aspect of reality. Within individuals, there can be no dysfunction unless it serves some function; analyzing individual components of a system is useful only if each component is related to the whole. Identification and placement in the correct behavioral and environmental context is also necessary to fully understand behavior. From a dialectic perspective, self-mutilation may be viewed as a "saving" event that enables patients to feel they can cope with life demands; it is also a destructive event contributing to depression, shame, suicide risk, and longer-term decreased coping.

A biosocial theory provides the primary lens for understanding how self-mutilation and other dysfunctional behaviors associated with BPD are developed and maintained. Within this perspective, individual dysfunction is regarded as extreme vulnerability to emotional dysregulation, whereas behavioral patterns such as self-mutilation arise from systemic dysregulation of primary emotions. Such dysregulation is the result of an ongoing transaction between individuals with varying degrees of biologically based difficulty in regulating emotion and environments that to varying degrees invalidate that individual's responses to the world. Invalidating environments are characterized by a tendency to disregard emotional experiences (particularly negative ones), to place a high value on positive thinking, and to oversimplify the ease of solving difficult problems.

Communications of nonpublic events and difficulties meeting social expectations are often not taken seriously in these vulnerable individuals. Such invalidating environments, especially those involving physical and sexual abuse, contribute to emotional dysregulation and fail to teach appropriate labeling of emotional experience, regulation of arousal, tolerance of emotional distress, and trust in one's own emotional experiences. The accumulation of such dysregulation and the inability to discern, trust, and accurately evaluate emotional experience are naturally self-reinforcing. DBT attributes the development and continued maintenance of BPD behavioral patterns to the incompatible transaction between this biologic vulnerability to emotion dysregulation and an invalidating environment.

## Treatment Stages and Targets

There are four stages in DBT, a pretreatment stage and three discrete treatment stages. An hierarchy of DBT targets determines the treatment agenda within and across sessions; each individual session agenda is set based on the client's behavior since the last session. It is the therapist's responsibility to remain mindful of treatment goals and to ensure that client activities are pointed in the direction of creating a life worth living.

In *pretreatment*, the patient is orientated to the philosophy and structure of DBT with the goal of making an agreement or commitment to pursue the goals of DBT. These goals are clearly prescribed. If a patient is currently engaging in parasuicide or self-mutilation, she must agree that reducing or eliminating such behavior is a goal to strive for: curtailing parasuicide of all types, including self-mutilation, is at all times the first priority. Patients must also agree not to kill themselves while they are in DBT. Although the dialectic coexistence of self-mutilation or other parasuicidal behavior and wishes to live is understood within DBT, treatment cannot progress beyond this target until these parasuicidal behaviors are under control. Obtaining explicit patient agreement is necessary prior to full participation in treatment; in settings in which patients may be reluctant to commit themselves to DBT goals, an ongoing pretreatment phase may be used to focus on commitment-enhancing strategies.

Stage 1 DBT targets life-threatening and suicidal behaviors, including parasuicide and self-mutilation. Forming and maintaining a good therapeutic relationship with a strong connection to the therapist and establishing stability are also primary targets. The targets during this stage include 1) decreasing self-harm, suicidal, or homicidal behaviors; 2) decreasing therapy-interfering behaviors, 3) decreasing quality of life–interfering behaviors; and 4) increasing the behavioral skills needed to make life changes—i.e., core mindfulness skills (the ability to focus thought and thinking), distress tolerance, emotion regulation skills, and interpersonal effectiveness skills.

Weekly diary cards are used to collect ongoing information about target problems. Targets are added to those listed on standard diary cards as needed but always include parasuicide (including self-mutilation); suicidal ideation and urges; prescription, licit, and illicit drug abuse; binge eating; general misery level; and a checklist to indicate DBT skills used during the week. These cards are reviewed at the beginning of each individual session, and the presence or absence of target problems since the last session identifies priorities for that session agenda. Self-monitoring via diary cards has several advantages over traditional memory-based narrative recall of events. It provides a source of feedback and data to the client and therapist that is unavailable through other means, and it may increase the accuracy of reported events. Structurally, the cards provide specific detail about the timing and relationship between self-mutilation and other dysfunctional behaviors and daily fluctuations in anxious or depressed mood, for example, intensity of anxious or depressed mood tied to self-mutilation, the level of mood that can be tolerated without resorting to self-mutilation, and so on.

Any direct self-harm; suicide crisis behavior; intrusive and intense suicidal ideation, images, or communications; or significant changes in suicidal ideation or urges to self-destruct are addressed in individual therapy immediately after their occurrence. Self-mutilation or other parasuicide behavior is never ignored. As good predictors of future lethal acts, these behaviors can cause substantial harm and, as primary targets, must be addressed before treatment can progress.

Stage 2 DBT addresses posttraumatic stress and invalidating experiences and may include processing and reexperiencing past trauma or emotionally important events. This does not occur, however, until the targets of Stage 1 are under control. A strong and capable commitment to being alive and the basic skills necessary to cope with dysregulation are regarded as prerequisites to entering Stage 2. Although patients might enter Stage 2 with suicidal ideation and strong wishes to be dead, they are not in Stage 2 if they are self-mutilating, buying guns for suicide, hoarding pills, or making other concrete plans. If Stage 1 may be thought of as guiding the patient to a state of quiet desperation (beginning from one of loud desperation), then Stage 2 raises the patient from unremitting emotional desperation (Koerner and Linehan 1997). Stage 3 treatment targets self-respect and achievement of individual goals through synthesis of prior DBT learning tasks. Developing an ongoing sense of connection to self, others, and to life is important as patients work toward resolving problems in living.

## Individual Treatment Strategies

The treatment strategies for DBT are conceptually divided into those related to acceptance and those related to change. There are four fundamental sets of treatment strategies that remain conceptually intact across all applications of DBT: 1) dialectical strategies, 2) core strategies (validation and problem solving), 3) communication strategies (irreverent and reciprocal communication), and 4) case management strategies (consultation with the patient, environmental intervention, and supervision/consultation with therapists) (see Table 7–1).

The DBT practitioner tries to balance the use of acceptance and change strategies within each treatment interaction. For example, behavior such as mutilation may prove to be both appropriate and valid because it may provide immediate relief from emotional pain or anxiety. At the same time, this behavior is highly dysfunctional and in need of change.

*Dialectical Strategies*

Dialectical strategies are best described as the struggle to balance acceptance of patients as they are now with the production of and movement toward change. As both a world view on the nature of reality and a change process, dialectics provide the framework for the synthesis of biologic and environmental approaches to the etiology and maintenance of BPD. Change occurs through the active synthesis of opposing forces; dialectical strategies emphasize balance and helping patients find reality in shades other than black and white. Increasing patients' comfort with inconsistency, ambiguity, and change is an important aim. By admitting and accepting incompatible realities as necessary, traditional behavior therapy methods are joined with acceptance of a fuller, often more realistic, perspective. Using stories, metaphors, and philosophy, dialectical strategies can be used to promote change or acceptance. Typical metaphors include those illustrating the difficulty of pursuing treatment ("like climbing out of hell on an aluminum ladder"), of accepting responsibility for pursuing help ("if you were hit by a car and broke your leg, would you refuse to have it set because it wasn't your fault the car hit you?"), and of acknowledging personal risk ("getting into your own warm bed with a poisonous snake, hoping against hope it will be asleep and won't bite you").

*Validation Strategies*

Validation strategies begin with empathy and extend to analyzing the patient's response in relationship to its context and function. There are three types of validation: verbal (direct communication that a statement is valid, e.g., "Yes, I can see that you're really upset"), functional (behavioral response that indicates the therapist accepts the client's statement as valid, e.g., "Let's take a look at what's upsetting you"), and cheerleading (validating individual capacity, not necessarily beliefs, e.g., client says "I can't

**Table 7-1.** Steps in behavioral (chain) analysis

1. Operational description of target problem behavior; detail overt behavior, verbalizations, cognitions, and affect, including intensity of the feelings

   **Example:**

   Overt behavior: located razor blade wrapped in tissue and stored in bottom of sock drawer; undressed and went into shower with razor; with water running, made a series of horizontal cuts across right wrist and forearm. Cuts were progressively deeper.

   Verbal: when mother knocked on door and asked, "What are you doing?" replied "Getting clean."

   Cognition: I deserve this, I need to do this, then reports she "stopped thinking."

   Affect: anxious (8=intensity); angry at self for being stupid (7), shame (9)

2. Specific precipitating event that began the chain, starting with environmental events (e.g., "Why did the problem occur yesterday rather than the day before?"

   **Example:**

   Patient went to see movie *Titanic* with cousin and aunt. Was very emotional throughout movie; felt it somehow was about her life. Afterwards, as they were discussing movie, tried to convey how important movie felt to her, felt ineffective, misunderstood, and thought they made fun of her for taking a movie so seriously.

3. Vulnerability-enhancing factors present (e.g., physical illness, poor sleeping, drug or alcohol abuse, or intense emotions)

   **Example:**

   Patient did not sleep well night before; had not eaten properly past 2–3 days—trying to diet, but bingeing and eating junk because holiday foods and sweets "around all the time." Feeling vulnerable emotionally because of holiday expectations, missing old boy-friend.

4. Detail moment-by-moment chain of events, examining thoughts, feelings, and actions; determine whether any possible alternatives were available

**Table 7–1.**  Steps in behavioral (chain) analysis *(continued)*

5. Identify consequences of problem behavior

   **Example:**

   Patient felt better, more in control, as though things had been set right and she could go to bed. Also felt stupid, has sabotaged treatment progress by allowing herself to "indulge" in self-mutilation. Felt she will disappoint therapist.

6. Generate alternative solutions—what skills might the client have used to avoid the problem behavior as a solution?

   **Examples:**

   Call therapist

   Review plans for these occasions

   Use distress tolerance skills

7. Identify a prevention strategy to reduce future vulnerability to problem chain

   **Example:**

   Anticipate, think about realistic interpersonal expectations of others. When I share with others who are not as sensitive as I am, what is my priority? That is, should/do I want to expect them to understand and be disappointed by their reaction?

8. Repair significant consequences of problem behavior through cheerleading, reducing vulnerability, reaffirming commitment

do it" and therapist replies, "I know you think you can't do it, but I have complete faith that you really can do it"). The function of validation is to make the unreasonable reasonable and to help patients learn how and when to trust themselves. Validation can also serve as acceptance to balance change and can function to strengthen clinical progress and the therapeutic relationship.

Validation is further broken down into six levels. Level 1, *active observing*, is unbiased listening and observing. Level 2, *reflecting the observed*, is an accurate reflection of and discussion about the identification, description, and labeling of client behavioral patterns. Level 3, *articulating the unobserved*, is articulating thoughts, memories, assumptions, and feelings that the patient is not verbalizing or expressing directly. Level 4, *validation in terms of the past or of biology*, is identifying the learning experiences and/ or biologic factors that make the patient's current responses inevitable while still identifying the behavior as dysfunctional in the moment. Level 5, *validation in terms of the present*, is identifying events in the current environment that produce current response patterns that make sense or are functional or normal response patterns. Level 6, *radical genuineness*, is treating the individual as valid. The task is to see and respond to the patient's strengths and capacities while remaining empathic toward actual difficulty and incapacity. For therapists, this involves throwing off preconceptions of patient role and acting fully, completely, and spontaneously— treating the patient as a person without role, not as fragile or invalid (mostly conveyed through voice tone). A therapist's condescending behavior, as felt by the patient, is often perceived as invalidating at level six, although it may be validating at levels 4 and 5.

### Problem-Solving Strategies

Based on the primary assumption that the lives of individuals with BPD are currently unbearable, DBT places great emphasis on change. DBT problem-solving strategies address each instance of parasuicide or other major dysfunctional behavior. Behavioral analysis is the most important method used for analyzing and understanding dysfunctional behavior because it provides the framework for generating solutions to such behavior. Behavioral analysis identifies the problem (self-mutilation), the preceding events and context (antecedents, conditioned cues, precipitant events, internal and external), and the events following the problem (consequences that may influence the behavior). A "chain" analysis is a very precise behavioral analysis of a single instance of a problem that results in a detailed step-by-step description of the precipitating events and the patient's emotional, cognitive, and overt behaviors that preceded the problem behavior. Finally,

**Table 7–2.** Dialectical behavior therapy procedures and strategies

| Acceptance | Change |
|---|---|
| 1. Dialectical | 1. Dialectical |
| 2. Validation | 2. Problem solving* |
| 3. Relationship | 3. Contingency management |
| 4. Environmental intervention | 4. Capability enhancement/skills acquisition |
| 5. Reciprocal communication | 5. Cognitive modification |
| | 6. Exposure |
| | 7. Consultation with the client |
| | 8. Irreverent communication |

*Includes behavioral analysis, insight/interpretation, solution analysis, didactic, trouble-shooting, and commitment strategies.

the consequences of engaging in the dysfunctional actions for both the client and the environment are examined. Once the chain of antecedents, behaviors, and consequences is clarified, the task becomes solution analysis—identifying how the basic change strategies can ameliorate the problem. Skills training addresses the patient's inability to engage in more adaptive responses; contingency management strategies address reinforcement strategies that support problematic behavior; cognitive modification procedures address faulty beliefs and assumptions that interfere with problem-solving capabilities; and exposure-based strategies address anxiety, shame, or other emotional responses that interfere with adaptive problem-solving attempts. Behavioral analysis may comprise a portion or even the entirety of a session. Table 7–2 illustrates a basic behavioral analysis.

Problem-solving procedures such as skills training, contingency management, cognitive modification, and exposure are adopted directly from the cognitive-behavioral literature. Patient and clinician together identify public and private problematic behaviors and factors associated with the initiation and maintenance of these problem patterns. Next, the behavioral excesses and deficits that interfere with the client's ability to engage in goal behaviors are identified, followed by what the patient must learn, experience, and do to perform the goal behavior.

### Exposure Strategies

Based on the important associations described earlier between shame and self-mutilation, change strategies using nonreinforced exposure to fear or emotions unwarranted in current situations are particularly salient in treating self-mutilation. As described by others (Foa and Rothbaum 1998; Resick and Schnicke 1993; Steketee 1993), basic exposure procedures include: 1) presenting stimuli that elicit the emotion; 2) providing corrective information so that the affective response is not reinforced; 3) blocking escape and other avoidance; and 4) enhancing the patient's sense of self-control. Functionally, three commonly used exposure strategies are 1) discussing and commenting on fear cues in a matter-of-fact or nonjudgmental manner; 2) discussing in detail the antecedents eliciting fear or anxiety (i.e., conducting a behavioral analysis); and 3) discussing in detail the ultimate feared consequences (catastrophes) of the feared situations.

Common fear cues and the therapist behaviors or events that elicit these topics encountered in DBT include the following:

- Fear of failure or of disappointing others; expectation of failures at tasks important to the patient and highlighting such failure
- Fear of being disliked; criticism or confrontation of a patient's dysfunctional behavior
- Fear of success (implying potential withdrawal of help and/or eventual failure); demands or expectations that the patient can do things that she says are impossible or that she might succeed
- Fear of losing control; linked to the belief that the patient is not and cannot actually be in control
- Fear of existential aloneness or of being more alone than is wanted
- Fear of not being loved or being rejected based on the fact that the therapeutic relationship is a professional relationship, not a friendship

In Stage 1 DBT, there is no formal protocol or procedure for using exposure strategies, and uncovering or reexposing patients to past trauma is avoided. Informally, exposure strategies are used to decrease emotional responses to present traumatic cues (e.g., loud noises, darkness, men) and to increase tolerance to current negative emotions (e.g., anger, shame). Particularly useful in treating the dissociative behavior often linked to self-mutilation are the skills of mindfulness and emotion regulation (described below), which are paired with exposure strategies. In some patients, particularly those whose trauma cues are related to more direct cues such as memories of past trauma or those who reexperience symptoms of trauma, the formal use of exposure to the actual traumatic experiences is required as part of Stage 2 DBT. The patient is presented with memories, thoughts, emotions, or events that elicit the response related to the traumatic experience (Wagner and Linehan, in press).

*Skills Training*

In DBT it is assumed that many of the problems experienced by patients who self-mutilate are caused by a combination of motivational problems and behavioral skill deficits—that is, the necessary skills to regulate painful affect were never originally learned. For this reason, DBT emphasizes skills building to facilitate behavior change and acceptance. In standard DBT, skills are taught weekly in 2.5-hour psychoeducational training groups. These skills are outlined and described in detail in the *Skills Training Manual for Borderline Personality Disorder* (Linehan 1993b). Individuals are taught specific behavioral skills necessary to ameliorate mutilation and other individual dysfunctional behavior patterns. Groups use a standard behavioral skills-building format and procedures, including modeling, instructions, behavioral rehearsal, feedback and coaching, and homework assignments.

Group skills training works in tandem with individual therapy. Simultaneous group and individual treatments create dedicated time to learn much-needed skills and a separate context for coached individual application. Clients with BPD frequently arrive for individual sessions in crisis and because the therapist typically attends to these issues, little time is left to learn skills. When skills are taught in group, the individual therapist can deal with current crises and also serve as a skills coach, encouraging transfer and generalization of particular skills. The group format has several advantages over individual skills training: participants learn from each other and practice skills with others engaged in the same tasks; skills practice coaching and feedback are available for a variety of members' responses; and group membership often decreases isolation and increases clients' sense of connection. The cotherapist role may be used and discussed as an interpersonal model. Socially phobic patients or those who must begin skills training in individual sessions are moved to group skills training as soon as possible. The four DBT skills training modules directly target the behavioral, emotional, and cognitive instability and dysregulation of BPD: mindfulness, interpersonal effectiveness, emotion regulation, and distress tolerance. In standard DBT, the first 2 weeks of any given module are spent on mindfulness and the remaining 6 weeks are spent on the particular module.

*Mindfulness* is a psychologic and behavioral translation of meditation skills usually taught in Eastern spiritual practices. The goals of this module are attentional control, awareness, and sense of true self. Three primary states of mind are presented: reasonable mind (the logical, analytical, problem-solving), emotion mind (the creative, passionate, and dramatic), and wise mind (the integration of both reasonable and emotion mind). Wise mind involves intuition and knowing what is right beyond reasoning and beyond direct experience. This synthesis of reasonable mind and emotion mind enables appropriate response; one responds as needed given the situation.

Group members first learn only to observe and then later to describe external and internal stimuli. Self-mutilation is regarded as a response of emotion mind—that is, although the results may feel positive in the short-term, they are negative in the longer term and lead to other painful states or events. Particularly among individuals with impulse control difficulty and those who use drugs or alcohol, acknowledging and labeling affective states is a major goal. Fully entering experiences, or participation, is the next mindfulness skill. Finally, patients learn that these acts are most useful when performed nonjudgmentally, one-mindfully, and effectively. Although these may sound like lofty Zen goals for patient mindfulness, the basic principles are expressed simply for learning and practice.

*Distress tolerance* focuses on the ability to accept both oneself and the current environmental situation in a nonevaluative manner. It is particularly useful for situations in which nothing can be immediately done to change the environment, such as with the patient who, when alone in her apartment at 3 AM, begins thinking the distressing series of thoughts that generally lead to self-mutilation but who does not want to engage in the behavior. Although implying acceptance of reality, distress tolerance does not imply approval. Activity-oriented distraction for improving the moment, sensory self-soothing, and consideration of the advantages and disadvantages of distress tolerance are skills within this module.

*Interpersonal effectiveness* skills are similar to standard interpersonal problem-solving and assertion training (Bower and Bower 1991). These skills include effective strategies for asking for what one needs and for saying "no" to requests. Effectiveness here is obtaining changes or objectives one wants, keeping the relationship, and building and maintaining self-respect. Developing clarity about expected and reasonable outcomes of interpersonal situations is a challenging task for many patients. As part of improving skills, the development of strategies and procedures for analyzing and planning interpersonal situations and for anticipating outcomes can decrease emotional vulnerability.

*Emotion regulation* is defined as the ability to 1) increase or decrease physiologic arousal associated with emotion; 2) reorient attention; 3) inhibit mood-dependent actions; 4) experience emotions without escalating or blunting; and 5) organize behavior in the service of external non–mood-dependent goals. This process begins with identifying and labeling current emotions by observing and describing events that prompt emotions; interpretating these events; and understanding the physiologic responses, emotionally expressive behaviors, and aftereffects of emotions. Reducing vulnerability to emotional reactivity and decreasing emotional suffering is also targeted. The focus on describing, labeling, and understanding primary emotional states is followed by strategies for reducing vulnerability to biologic needs and steps for increasing positive emotions. A patient identifies the emotions that precipitate her self-mutilation, explores their function, and learns to monitor her specific vulnerabilities (e.g., sleep, eating, alcohol or drug use) and to build in positive, pleasant, goal-oriented, competence-enhancing experiences that strengthen her resistance to the emotion mind that precedes self-mutilation.

Although the above skills are taught as independent skills sets, the avoidance of repetitive dysfunctional behavior such as self-mutilation may involve use of two or more skills as determined by the individual's behavioral chain leading to the event.

### Communication and Stylistic Strategies

*Reciprocal communication* is characterized by genuineness, warm engagement, and responsiveness. Responsiveness requires the therapist to take patients' agendas and wishes seriously and to respond directly to the content of their communications rather than interpreting or suggesting that the content or intent of these communications is invalid. The use of self-involving self-disclosures, such as pointing out the effects of the patient's behavior on the therapist in a nonjudgmental manner, and of personal self-disclosures, which are used to validate and model coping and normative responses, are encouraged. *Irreverent communication* involves a direct, confrontational, matter-of-fact, or "off-the-wall" style. Used to help move the patient from a rigid stance to one that admits uncertainty, irreverent communication is highly useful when therapist and patient are stuck or at an impasse. Irreverence may be attained when the therapist pays closer attention to the patient's indirect rather than direct communications. For example, when a patient says, "I am going to kill myself," the therapist might irreverently respond, "But I thought you agreed not to drop out of therapy." Care is taken in observing the effects of irreverent communication, to avoid misuse and potentially alienating the patient.

### Supervision and Consultation

Dialectical behavior therapy is best applied as a treatment system in which the therapist applies DBT to patients while the supervisor or consultation team simultaneously apply DBT to the therapist. Consultation with the therapist serves several functions: most importantly, ensuring the clinician remains in the therapeutic relationship and remains effectively in that relationship. Without ongoing supervision or consultation, clinicians working with this patient population can become extreme in their positions, blame the patient and themselves, and become less open to feedback from others about the conduct of their treatment.

## Telephone Consultation

Contact between sessions is an integral component of DBT and serves three functions: 1) coaching in skills and promoting skills generalization; 2) emergency crisis intervention in a contingent manner; and 3) an opportunity to resolve misunderstandings and conflicts that arise during therapy sessions instead of waiting until the next session to deal with such emotions. Typical skills coaching situations include those when the patient is not certain which skill to use or feels the skill is inhibited. DBT clients are typically invited to call before suicidal crises, or at least before they harm themselves. Consistent with the therapist's role as coach for adaptive behavior, this contact must occur before the self-mutilation or other parasuicidal behavior; if the patient has already engaged in self-mutilation, the "24-hour rule" stipulates that patients cannot have supportive phone contact with the therapist for 24 hours after parasuicide and phone contact is limited to management only. This provides reinforcement for adaptive coping and realistic consequences after the fact—"What help can I give you after you've already decided to hurt yourself?"

## Environmental Components: Casework and Consultation

Case management or environmental intervention strategies are the least developed component of standard DBT but contain strategies critical to skills generalization: patients learn self-advocacy, and therapists perform casework activities only when the patient lacks the skill and cannot learn it quickly enough to prevent an immediately adverse outcome from occurring. DBT's strong learning theory orientation applies case management strategies differently than traditionally described in the case management literature. The skills building focus fosters belief in the clients' ability to learn more effective ways of intervening in their own environments. Advocacy for its own sake is not regarded as an empowering or helpful act. Direct environmental intervention by the therapist is approved only under certain conditions, including 1) when the client is unable to act on her own and the outcome is very important (e.g., the suicidal, depersonalizing client who cannot to tell her family she needs them to stay with her); 2) when the environment is intransigent and high in power (e.g., an application for social services that requires professional involvement); 3) to save the life of the client or to avoid substantial risk to others (e.g., high suicidality or risk of child abuse); 4) when it is the humane thing to do and will cause no harm—that is, does not substitute passive for active problem solving (e.g., meeting with client outside ordinary setting in a crisis); and 5) when the client is a minor.

DBT case management helps clients manage their physical and social environments to enhance overall life functioning and well-being. Case management strategies include consultation with the patient, environmental intervention, and therapist supervision/consultation. These function as guidelines for applying the DBT core strategies to the environment outside the client–therapist relationship. The therapist coaches the client on effective interaction with the environment and works to generalize skills. If the client does not possess the requisite skill for effectively intervening in the environment and the situation requires immediate resolution, the therapist acts as advocate and model, interacting with other professionals on behalf of the client, but only in the client's presence.

Marital and family involvement was originally limited to consultation with the patient about how to handle family and friends; others were not actively involved in DBT. Consultation helps the client communicate effectively with her family about treatment and about needs from friends and family. Conflict resolution and problem solving are also frequently part of consultation. Family sessions are held if client and therapist agree they would be useful, but never without the client.

In response to high distress on the part of the families of BPD clients, and in an effort to more directly access this important aspect of the client's environment, recent adaptations of DBT have included direct family involvement. Fruzetti et al. (in press) have extended DBT to the families and significant others of patients with BPD. DBT for families contains both psychoeducational didactic and skills building components. Families meet in multiple-family groups or in individual sessions, generally with the patient present. The biosocial model of BPD is explained and the characteristics of BPD are identified and normalized. Families learn DBT skills to help support clients in their efforts to change and also to help themselves cope with the patients' dysfunctional behavior patterns. Mindfulness, distress tolerance, interpersonal effectiveness, and emotion regulation are taught in similar fashion to their presentation in the skills manual.

## Summary and Future Directions in Treatment

Dialectical behavior therapy is an empirically derived treatment for parasuicide, including self-mutilation, and other characteristic behaviors associated with BPD. It is humane and incorporates a biosocial perspective, acknowledging the powerful role of the environment in the etiology and maintenance of these often longstanding behavioral patterns. DBT has demonstrated effectiveness in two randomized clinical trials treating women with BPD, and less-controlled studies suggest that promising adaptations are developing. As development and adaptation of DBT to other problems and settings occurs, it is important that those conducting these efforts remain clear about the need to continue essential empirical validation of this treatment. Efforts to more specifically target and classify self-mutilation make up a significant focus of DBT development and investigation.

## References

American Psychological Association: Task Force on Promotion and Dissemination of Psychological Procedures: A Report Adopted by the Division 12 Board. Washington, DC, American Psychological Association, 1993

Anderson L: Notes on the linkage between the sexually abused child and the suicidal adolescent. Journal of Adolescence 4:157–162, 1981

Bach-Y-Rita G: Habitual violence and self-mutilation. Am J Psychiatry 131:1018–1029, 1974

Barley WD, Buie SE, Peterson EW, et al: The development of an inpatient cognitive-behavioral treatment program for borderline personality disorder. J Personal Disord 7:232–240, 1993

Bower SA, Bower GH: Asserting Yourself: A Practical Guide for Positive Change. New York, Addison-Wesley, 1991

Brown M, Linehan MM: The relationship between negative emotions and parasuicide in borderline personality disorder. Presented at Association for Advancement of Behavior Therapy annual convention, New York, November 1996

Brown M, Levensky E, Linehan MM: The relationship between shame and parasuicide in borderline personality disorder. Presented at Association for Advancement of Behavior Therapy annual convention, Miami Beach, FL, November 1997

Endicott J, Spitzer RL, Fleiss JL, et al: The Global Assessment Scale. Arch Gen Psychiatry 33:766–771, 1976

Favazza A: Why patients mutilate themselves. Hospital and Community Psychiatry 40:137–145, 1989

Favazza A, Conterio K: Female habitual self-mutilators. Acta Psychiatr Scand 79:283–289, 1989

Foa EB, Rothbaum BO: Treating the Trauma of Rape Cognitive-Behavioral Therapy for PTSD. New York, Guilford, 1998

Frances AJ, Fyer MR, Clarkin JF: Personality and suicide. Ann N Y Acad Sci 487:281–293, 1986

Freud A: Aggression in Relation to Emotional Development in the Psychoanalytic Study of the Child. New York, Universities Press, 1949

Fruzetti AE, Hoffman PD, Linehan MM: Dialectical Behavior Therapy with Couples and Families. New York, Guilford, in press

Fyer MR: Suicide attempts in patients with borderline personality disorder. Am J Psychiatry 145:737–739, 1988

Gardner AR, Gardner AJ: Self-mutilation obessionality and narcissism. Br J Psychiatry 127:127–132, 1975

Gardner DL, Cowdry RW: Suicidal and parasuicidal behavior in borderline personality. Psychiatry Clin North Am 8:389–403, 1985

Graff H, Mallin R: The syndrome of the wrist cutter. Am J Psychiatry 127:127–132, 1967

Greenspan GS, Samuel SE: Self-cutting after rape. Am J Psychiatry 146:789–790, 1989

Gunderson JG: Borderline Personality Disorder. Washington, DC, American Psychiatric Press, 1984

Haines J, Williams C, Brian K, et al: The psychophysiology of self-mutilation. J Abnorm Psychol 104:479–489, 1996

Hillbrand M, Krystal J, Sharpe K, et al: Clinical predictors of self-mutilation in hospitalized forensic patients. J Nerv Ment Dis 182:9–13, 1994

Ivanoff A, Smyth NJ, Grochowski S, et al: Problem solving and suicidality among prison inmates. J Consult Clin Psychol 60:970–973, 1992

Jones A: Self-mutilation in prison: a comparison of mutilators and nonmutilators. Criminal Justice and Behavior 13:286–296, 1986

Jones IH, Congin L, Stevenson J, et al: A biological approach to two forms of human self–injury. J Nerv Ment Dis 167:74–78, 1979

Kaplan H, Pokorny A: Self-derogation and psychosocial adjustment. J Nerv Ment Dis 149:421–434, 1969

Kehrer CA, Linehan MM: Interpersonal and emotional problem solving skills and parasuicide among women with borderline personality disorder. J Personal Disord 10:153–163, 1996

Kemperman I, Russ M, Shearin EN: Self-injurious behavior and mood regulation in borderline patients. J Personal Disord 11:146–157, 1997

Koerner K, Linehan MM: Case formulation in dialectical behavior therapy for borderline personality disorder, in Handbook of Psychotherapy Case Formulation. Edited by Eells T. New York, Guilford, 1997, pp 340–367

Kreitman N: Parasuicide. London, England, John Wiley and Sons, 1977

Leibenluft E, Gardner DL, Cowdry RW: The inner experience of the borderline self-mutilator. J Personal Disord 1:317–324, 1987

Liebowitz MR: A medication approach. J Personal Disord 1:325–327, 1987

Linehan MM: A social-behavioral analysis of suicide and parasuicide: implications for clinical assessment and treatment, in Depression: Behavioral and Directive Intervention Strategies. Edited by Glazer H, Clarkin JF. New York, Garland, 1981, pp 229–294

Linehan MM: Cognitive-Behavioral Treatment for Borderline Personality Disorder. New York, Guilford, 1993a

Linehan MM: Skills Training Manual for Treating Borderline Personality Disorder. New York, Guilford, 1993b

Linehan MM: Behavioral treatment of suicidal behaviors: definitional obfuscation and treatment outcomes, in Neurobiology of Suicide: From the Bench to the Clinic. Edited by Stoff DM, Mann JJ. New York, Annals of the New York Academy of Sciences, 1997a, pp 302–328

Linehan MM: Validation and psychotherapy, in Empathy Reconsidered: New Directions in Psychotherapy. Edited by Bohart A, Greenberg L. Washington, DC, American Psychological Association, 1997b, pp 353–392

Linehan MM, Heard HL: Impact of treatment accessibility on clinical course of parasuicidal patients: reply to R.E. Hoffman (letter to editor). Arch Gen Psychiatry 50:157–158, 1993

Linehan MM, Camper P, Chiles JA, et al: Interpersonal problem solving and parasuicide. Cognitive Therapy and Research 11:1–12, 1987

Linehan MM, Armstrong HE, Suarez A, et al: Cognitive-behavioral treatment of chronically parasuicidal borderline patients. Arch Gen Psychiatry 48:1060–1064, 1991

Maris R: Pathways to Suicide: A Survey of Self-Destructive Behaviors. Baltimore, MD,The Johns Hopkins University Press, 1981

Miller A, Rathus JH, Linehan MM, et al: Dialectical behavior therapy adapted for suicidal adolescents. J Pract Psychiatry Behav Health 3:78–86, 1997

Morgan HG: Death Wishes? Chichester, England, Wiley, 1979

Pao PE: The syndrome of delicate self-cutting. Br J Med Psychol 42:195–206, 1969

Pattison EM, Kahan J: The deliberate self-harm syndrome. Am J Psychiatry 140:867–872, 1983

Resick PA, Schnicke MK: Cognitive Processing Therapy for Rape Victims: A Treatment Manual. Newbury Park, CA, Sage Publications, 1993

Rosenthal RJ, Rinzler C, Walsh R, et al: Wrist-cutting syndrome: the meaning of a gesture. Am J Psychiatry 128:1363–1368, 1972

Ross R, McKay H, Palmer W, et al: Self-mutilation in adolescent female offenders. Canadian Journal of Criminology 20 375–392, 1978

Roy A: Self-mutilation. Br J Med Psychol 51:201–203, 1978

Schotte DE, Clum GA: Problem-solving skills in suicidal psychiatric patients. J Consult Clin Psychol 55:49–54, 1987

Shapiro S: Self-mutilation and self-blame in incest victims. Am J Psychother 41:46–54, 1987

Shneidman ES: A psychological approach to suicide, in Cataclysms, Crises, and Catastrophes: Psychology in Action. The Master Lectures. Edited by VandenBos GR, Bryant BK. Washington, DC, American Psychological Association, 1987, pp 147–183

Simeon D, Stanley B, Frances A, et al: Self-mutilation in personality disorders: psychological and biological correlates. Am J Psychiatry 149:221–226, 1992

Simpson MA: Self-mutilation and suicide, in Suicidology: Contemporary Developments. Edited by Shneidman ES. New York, Grune and Stratton, 1976

Steketee GS: Treatment of Obsessive-Compulsive Disorder. New York, Guilford, 1993

Stone MH, Hurt SW, Stone DK: The PI 500: long-term follow-up of borderline inpatients meeting DSM-III criteria, I: Global outcome. J Personal Disord 1:291–298, 1987

Swenson C, Sanderson C, Linehan MM: Applying dialectical behavior therapy on inpatient units, in press

Telch CF: Skills training treatment for adaptive affect regulation in a woman with binge-eating disorder. Int J Eat Disord 22:77–81, 1997

Wagner AW, Linehan MM: The relationship between childhood sexual abuse and suicidal behaviors in borderline patients, in The Role of Sexual Abuse in the Etiology of Borderline Personality Disorder. Edited by Zanarini M. Washington, DC, American Psychiatric Association, 1997, pp 203–223

Wagner AW, Linehan MM: Dissociation, in Trauma in Context: A Cognitive-Behavioral Approach. Edited by Follette VM, Ruzek JI, Abueg FR. New York, Guilford, in press

Walsh BW: Adolescent self-mutilation: an empirical study (dissertation). Boston, MA, Boston College Graduate School of Social Work, 1987

Walsh BW, Rosen PM: Self-Mutilation: Theory, Research, and Treatment. New York, Guilford, 1988

Widiger TA, Frances AJ: Epidemiology diagnosis and comorbidity of borderline personality disorder, in American Psychiatric Press Review of Psychiatry, Vol 8. Edited by Tasman A, Hales RE, Frances AJ.Washington DC: American Psychiatry Press, 1987, pp 8–24

Widiger TA, Weissman MM: Epidemiology of borderline personality disorder. Hospital and Community Psychiatry 42:1015–1021, 1991

Wilkinson J, Coid J: Self-mutilation in female remanded prisoners, I: an indicator of severe psychopathology. Criminal Behavior and Mental Health 1:247–267, 1991

Winchel RM, Stanley M: Self-injurious behavior: a review of the behavior and biology of self-mutilation. Am J Psychiatry 148:306–317, 1991

# CHAPTER 8

# Psychodynamic Theory and Treatment of Impulsive Self-Injurious Behaviors

### Orna Guralnik, Psych.D.
### Daphne Simeon, M.D.

*T*he phenomenon of people inflicting pain and injury on themselves is complex and disturbing and confronts us with the potential depths of human despair. The conscious decision to harm oneself seems contrary to the basic premise that behaviors are intended to promote and better survival and is generally considered a sign of severe pathology. It demonstrates a brutal split within the self-mutilator into both an attacking agent and a victimized one. The destructiveness and agony involved in the act of self-mutilation and the challenge this act poses to basic premises about the unity and goal of self-determined behavior make it pressing yet difficult to understand and treat. The intense reactions that self-mutilation tends to evoke in others further complicate attempts to address it. These reactions include helplessness—the witness wants to protect the self-mutilator and stop the destructiveness of the act; rage at being helplessly left out of this drama within the person; and fear of empathizing or identifying with such destructive urges. Furthermore, it can be difficult to decipher the indirect communications such self-injurious actions imply.

In this chapter we review several central, psychodynamically informed approaches to impulsive self-injury in nonpsychotic or developmentally disabled people. Although behavior is multidetermined, for the sake of clarity these approaches are discussed separately. The goal is to inform clinicians of the main conceptualizations of self-injury in different theoretical frameworks. Generally, the theoretical approaches reviewed can be categorized into those that focus on the intrapsychic meanings of the behavior and those that focus on interpersonal determinants. More traditional psychoanalytic notions tend to formulate self-injury as a compromise formation in response to conflicts over libidinal and/or aggressive drives, whereas object relational theories focus on the playing out of battles between internalized self and object representations. From a self-psychologic perspective, self-mutilation can be understood as an attempt to consolidate the self, as a way of affirming one's boundaries, and as a self-soothing function. Interpersonal approaches assign meaning to behavior in the social context in which it emerges, and self-mutilation is understood as an act of communication between people: it may reflect a response to immediate circumstances or a belated reenactment of historical interpersonal matrixes.

If considered on their own, these different schools of thought may lead to drastically differing interventions. However, human behavior is highly complex and expressive of many layers of meaning, self-mutilation not withstanding. Simpson (1980) describes wrist cutting as "a supremely economical technique whereby a delicate dermal injury can serve multiple psychological functions in the cutter, while stirring up an inordinate amount of attention from others whose outrage and alarm is usually out of all proportion to the scale of the event" (p. 258). For proper management, the clinician's responsibility is to be open to hearing the patient's story, equipped with a wide and creative variety of interpretations and tools to intervene with, and able to use one's own reactions as an important source of information rather than as a distorting filter. Depending on the function of the behavior for the individual, its severity, and the patient's stage in treatment, management may include an emphasis on ego strengthening and limit setting, mirroring, containment of powerful affects, active interpretations, or articulation of the interpersonal impacts and meanings of the behaviors. We chose to focus on a selection of theoretical approaches to the understanding of self-mutilation and their treatment implications, followed by a discussion of countertransference and its management issues.

## Classical Approach

The classical psychoanalytic conceptualization of self-injurious behaviors (SIBs) generally views them as vicissitudes of instincts within the structural tripartite model of the mind; primitive drives threaten to overwhelm the ego and either find expression through acting out or are curtailed by the superego. Self-mutilation is seen as a direct expression of either aggressive or sexual drives or the fusion of both. A common interpretation sees self-injury as the turning of the primary instinct of aggression against the self, or as a manifestation of the primary death instinct that can be directed outward or redirected inward (Cooper 1988). Bennum (1983) explains self-mutilation as the individual's way of controlling powerful experiences of hostility and tension. Hostile impulses can be either channeled outward or inward ("intropunitive"). Bennum conducted a study comparing self-mutilators with nonmutilating depressed patients in which both groups were equally intropunitive and depressed in terms of severity. However, self-mutilators differed in a stronger degree of self-abasement and criticism, including guilt and self-punitiveness, whereas nonmutilators with depression loaded higher on vegetative components of depression. The self-mutilators were also higher on acting-out hostility and had poorer impulse control. According to Crabtree (1967), self-mutilation is a sadomasochistic autoperversion expressing a self-enclosed way of dealing with impulses, such that the patient takes his own body as a libidinal object. Thus, the behavior reflects narcissistic, autoerotic, and autoaggressive involvement. The sexual components of such behavior are supported by the rhythm of mounting anxiety and excitation before the act and the sense of relief, calm, and even happiness that follow.

A different angle sees self-mutilation as an expression of primitive and intolerable guilt in response to impulses. The guilt is hypothesized to be induced by either aggressive fantasies, such as mutilating fantasies against the parents, or primitive libidinal impulses. The self-mutilators' fierce self-denigration and intense guilt are reflective of a severe, relentless, primitive superego (Simpson 1980). Their self-mutilative actions are understood as direct expressions of the punitive functions of the primitive superego. Friedman et al. (1972) described self-mutilation as motivated by the pressure of regressive sexual incestuous fantasies that are felt to be constantly threatening to overwhelm the ego. The urges are not controlled and contained by fantasy and masturbation, but rather create a pressure to "live them out repetitively." Patients describe hating their bodies for feeling forced by their bodies to have fantasies and to act them out. Mutilation is therefore aimed at destroying the body as the source of urges. It differs from attempted suicide because it expresses an unconscious fantasy to destroy the genitals through displacement, whereas in suicide the whole body is attacked. The calm following the act is interpreted as a relief that the genitals remain safe. An additional function that has been suggested is that by attacking one's own body, the experience of helplessness in the face of aggressive and sexual urges is turned into one of omnipotent control (Friedman et al. 1972).

From a more ego-psychologic perspective focusing on adaptation, the underlying masochistic dynamics of self-mutilation can be understood as an act of self-preservation, a compromise between instinctual and repressive forces. Arons (1981) described the process of a person making an internal bargain to reduce or undo overwhelming guilt. A sense of wrongdoing, most likely Oedipal guilt, mobilizes an overly harsh and primitive conscience to retaliate. The guilt is symbolically condensed into a body part that becomes detached from the self and sacrificed in an act of self-punishment, allowing preservation of life. Feelings and actions are displaced from the genitals to other organs invested with sexual importance. It is a compromise formation that averts total annihilation or symbolic castration.

Modern Freudian approaches focus on self-mutilation as a form of regression to early states in which drives and a mostly somatic level of experience are manifested. The skin, being one of the first definers and mediators of the self, is central to the body ego. When the body ego functions are impaired, a diffuse instinctual anxiety emerges because the id is not being sufficiently contained. Self-cutting is a somatic playing-out of intolerable affects similar to those experienced in the earliest months of the infant, when all experiences were somatic occurrences.

## Implications for Treatment

Classical theories interpret self-mutilation as an expression of aggressive or sexual impulses or as the reaction of a harsh superego to forbidden impulses. The classical approach to treatment can be summarized as an ongoing effort to make the unconscious conscious and uncover the repressed impulses that lead to self-injury. By way of interpretation, the therapist helps the patient understand the underlying meaning of the behavior, make peace between different parts of the psyche, and develop more sophisticated defense mechanisms to negotiate between powerful impulses and the superego. The self-mutilating behavior is consistently interpreted as having symbolic meaning, with the idea that making the underlying sexual or aggressive pressures conscious will reduce the compulsion to act and allow for the development of more effective defenses. In fact, patients have reported that once they understood underlying motives to their self-mutilation, the behavior itself became less compelling (Kwawer 1980). Adding an ego-psychologic perspective, Bennum (1983) recommended simultaneously focusing on ego strengthening and developing impulse control methods while searching for alternative ways to defuse hostility.

## Object Relations Approach

Whereas classical psychoanalytic formulations focus on the vicissitudes of libidinal and aggressive strivings as well as superego pathology, a different frame of reference focuses on the organization and pathology of internalized object relations. The various mental representations of others encapsulate aspects of significant objects as well as the ways in which these objects were affectively experienced and related to by aspects of the subject. One of the important shifts that object relations theory offered to psychoanalytic thinking was a heightened awareness of the impact of early relationships as well as the crucial importance of fantasy. With its inherent split into attacking and victimized agents, self-mutilation easily lends itself to be interpreted as reflecting struggles and negotiations between different self and object representations. The aggressiveness of the behavior marks an object world populated with critical persecutors and sparse in sources of internal security and resource.

Klein (1935/1986) described the process by which the ego marshals the same forces against internal prosecutors that it employs against those in the outside world. In the complex relationships between introjected objects, a self-injurious gesture can be seen as an act of the ego intending to murder its bad objects while saving the loved ones. Part of the ego, identified with the good internalized objects, is preserved while the parts identified with the bad objects and the id are attacked. Klein viewed suicidal gestures in part as struggles to protect one's good objects, ultimately the good mother, from the uncontrollably dangerous hatred and revenge that well up and threaten to sadistically attack them. The torturous experience of dependence on one's loved objects drives the ego to seek freedom but the identification with these objects is too profound to be renounced.

In a similar vein, self-mutilation has been studied as the product of a struggle against regressive pulls and aggressions toward the mother. This connection was explored by a group of British psychoanalysts that studied acts of self-mutilation and attempted suicides in a group of adolescent patients (Friedman et al. 1972). It is important to mention here that most nonpsychotic/autistic acts of self-mutilation first emerge in adolescence (Favazza 1989). These acts are explained by Friedman et al. (1972) as being determined by both primitive ties to the mother and alterations in the adolescent's relationship to his/her own body. A common theme that emerged in the treatment of the adolescent group members was their inability to give up strong ambivalent ties to their mothers, ties that included intense hostility. Internal moves toward breaking these ties threatened to result in unbearable loss of vital libidinal supplies. Rather than separating from the mother, she was retained through introjection. These narcissistic identifications were harshly and constantly attacked by the patients' relentless and severe superegos. Acts of self-mutilation were therefore interpreted as attacks on the internalized object—invariably the mother. The authors observed that on an overt level these patients demonstrated an "unremitting need not to give in to their mothers" (p. 181), which was viewed as a defense against the regressive passive wishes in relation to the mother. The defensive use of aggression against regressive wishes made it more difficult for these adolescents to control aggression. An example is the case of Sally, a 19-year-old woman who lost her mother at the age of 5 and began slashing her thighs and arms around puberty. Her attacks on herself were triggered by situations of longing, whereby she would get in touch with powerful cravings for her dead mother and experience her self-cutting as a way of symbolically bonding with her. Sally simultaneously experienced rage at her mother's unavailability and inability to respond to her needs as well as contempt toward her own longings, which gave a vicious spin to her attacks on herself. Focusing on aspects of mastery in the act of self-mutilation, Cooper (1988) understood self-mutilations as attempts to reinforce a sense of freedom from the need to cling that result in a sense of pleasure in the accomplishment of separation.

## Implications for Treatment

Object relational theories approach self-mutilation as the externalization of conflictual relationships between internalized objects and self-representations. Some theories emphasize attempts to sever difficult bonds and reach a sense of autonomy and mastery while trying to kill regressive/clingy needs. Interpretations from an object relational perspective emphasize patterns of relatedness and needs as they emerge and develop in early relationships and also make connections to transference reenactments. In addition to the goal of making the unconscious conscious, there is an attempt to clarify the historical and relational context to the patient's internal dynamics and develop the ability to know and express these forces in words. The transference/countertransference constellations serve as a data collecting arena as well as a practicing field for new relational patterns. An important aspect of this approach includes making explicit the existence of dependent and clingy needs, both in the transference and in relation to significant others, and clarifying the patient's intolerance of these needs. There is an attempt to clarify why such needs seem so threatening, considering one's history. In this context the attack on the self is often reframed as actually an attack on the other at one's own expense.

Part of what the object relational perspective offers to patients is a framework from which to make sense of their chaotic internal experiences. Patients learn to relate aspects of their experience to their history and to people in their lives and also learn to work through the primitive self-blaming and guilt they tend to feel for their destructive urges. As with any psychodynamically oriented treatment, having a story they can understand organizes the patients' experiences and drastically reduces their pressure to reenact.

## Approaches Focusing on the Self

In addition to increasing a sense of mastery over dependency strivings and strengthening a sense of separation from a frustrating or threatening mothering figure, self-mutilation may serve to enhance self-definition and to establish a clearer sense of boundaries. Focusing on the self-mutilator's attempt to form a coherent sense of self, Cooper (1988) discussed the gratifying and constructive aspects of self-inflicted pain sensations. Painful bodily (particularly skin) experiences are understood to be important proprioceptive mechanisms that assist in forming the body image and self-image. This is supported by those people who are relieved from body diffusion by inflicting pain to their skin (Favazza 1989; Kafka 1969). Skin sensations of all kinds, and especially moderately painful ones, are ways of achieving necessary and gratifying self-definition and boundaries. In the developmental process of separation and individuation, pain is a necessary concomitant of separation because it is a lesser evil than the damage and decay of the self that would result from failure of separation. Self-mutilation reflects the difficulty in establishing a clear body schema and integrating mental and bodily self. According to Rosiello (1993), self-inflicted pain and masochistic behavior serve to restore a sense of self via omnipotent narcissistic fantasies, including a sense of illusory control over infantile vulnerability by choosing to endure pain. It is performed for the sake of control and power in order to sustain a firmer self-cohesion. The masochistic experience includes fantasies of being pure and alone while renouncing the world and emerging triumphant.

A different angle relates SIBs to dissociative processes. Acts of self-mutilation can become a powerful tool to alter self-states. At least half of the patients that self-mutilate experience depersonalization and a sense of analgesia during the act (Leibenluft et al. 1987). Dissociation and depersonalization, although providing protection from overwhelming affect, result in a subjective sense of deadness, disconnection from others, and internal disintegration (van der Kolk et al. 1991). For some, the act provides a means of breaking this intolerable dissociative spell and feeling alive again. For others it is a way of inducing a more dissociative state in response to feeling overwhelmed and enhancing a dissociation of body from self.

Self-mutilation is an effective way to modulate intense affect, with some self-mutilators reporting it to be a mechanism to relieve them from dysphoria (Leibenluft et al. 1987). Others use it as a way of inducing euphoria and titillation (Favazza 1989; Simpson 1980). Self-mutilation also serves as a distraction from troubling thoughts and conflicts, such as preoccupations with abandonment or sexuality. Self-mutilation can thus serve a general self-regulatory function. Its organizing and distracting functions are reminiscent of addictive behaviors—the characteristic repetitive/ritualistic elements in the act, the internal struggle yet compulsion to perform, the cycle of mounting anxiety and relief, and the frequent development of "kits," such as self-cutting kits, that include elaborate paraphernalia. Similar to substance abusers, self-mutilators often exhibit a pattern of reacting with extremes of under- and overarousal to even minor emotional stressors, with stress responses that do not extinguish over time. They share similar patterns of addiction to the dramatic cycles of arousal and relief and an acquired numbness and insensitivity to more subtle emotional experiences that do not cross their sensation threshold. They often seem not to notice or ignore subtle internal and external events, and "wake up" to the world only when their internal state is overwhelming. In essence, SIBs become a quick and powerful method for self-regulation.

Related to its self-soothing function, some clinicians have noticed the transitional-object qualities self-mutilation can acquire for some people. Blood in particular is repeatedly described as a solacing transitional object (Favazza 1989). In a case study reported by Kafka (1969), self-injury was a way of making the patient's own body her transitional object. When the patient in this study described that slow and deliberate cutting of her skin to her therapist, she reported not feeling the cutting for a while and stopping as soon as the feeling of "becoming alive" set in. The blood gave her a sensation of pleasant warmth, like a potential security blanket she carried within herself. Kafka related the blood to the patient's internalized mother, with the patient feeling superior to others in her ability to generate this comforting mother-blanket at will.

## Implications for Treatment

Self-mutilation can become very stubborn and resistant to change, which accentuates the important function it must serve for the patient. Understanding SIB as a need to shore up a crumbling self implies the need for intense attunement in the treatment, particularly of split off and hidden aspects of the self that are involved in the masochistic activity. It is important to avoid interventions that are shaming or blaming to patients while using every chance to provide mirroring, containing, and self-enhancing interventions. Patients will remain unresponsive to outside influences as long as they remain in a state of psychic numbing. One of the ultimate goals of therapy would be to increase tolerance and capacity to regulate affect and to develop the process of thinking as a helpful way to process intense emotions. This includes intermediate steps along the way to relieve patients of tension and overwhelming affect, including the development of coping techniques and less destructive ways of distracting and distancing oneself. The therapeutic process involves several components that often follow each other, including 1) the *identification* of the feeling states, often manifested in extreme anxiety and tension, and the source of excitation. As described earlier, the tension is frequently triggered by anger and rage as well as by strong needs or longings, including sexual desires and even strivings for health or success. Patients often fail to make the connection between their internal state and the events that precipitated their feelings. The growing sense of tension is also often a response to threats to the patient's sense of self-cohesion or esteem. 2) Once identified, ways to care for oneself should be developed as alternatives to extreme patterns of excitation and numbness. This involves developing the ability to tolerate more tension and discomfort and the willingness to allow for a slower and more controlled pace of reducing discomfort. 3) Ways of negotiating with the environment are learned, an issue that will be further elaborated on in the interpersonal section of the chapter. These steps help moderate the extreme cycles of overreactivity in such patients.

To further elaborate on these components, in the process of developing distress tolerance, therapists need to educate patients about the existence of a self-soothing function that helps them get through situations that evoke distress. This concept often comes as a radically new idea to some patients. Exploring with patients their current ways of responding to internal states and developing new ways for dealing with their internal world can be surprisingly helpful. This process can include clarifying the importance of "talking to oneself" internally and of making organizing self-statements rather than the automatic self-derogatory and attacking internal dialogue usually present. Self-statements are a way of sensitizing patients to developing an internalized agent that assumes a caretaking role, for example, by explaining to oneself what is happening, what one might be feeling, and reminding oneself of prior plans made for stressful situations.

Over time, patients' sensitivity to nuances can develop, with a growing ability to prevent escalation into an overwhelmed or numb state. They can learn to think of relationships as a source of comfort and realize the benefits of making contact with others to help them with their feelings. Although a central part of their treatment will involve developing new ways of relating to others to achieve those goals, the development of impulse control is necessary to allow them to channel and defuse feelings, such as needs and hostility, within relationships. Patients will give up their old methods only if they have a new way of serving a similar function that will involve some sense of gratification. In this case, one of the immediate sources of gratification in changing is the sense of control and mastery. A long-term satisfaction comes from the developed ability to sort through feelings within the context of a relationship, which makes it deeper and more reliable.

## Role of Trauma in Impulsive Self-Injury

A key issue in the study of self-mutilation is its relation to histories of childhood trauma. Self-mutilators are frequently reported to have a history of developmental losses, unpredictable environments, and outright physical and sexual abuse in childhood (Leibenluft et al. 1987; Stone 1992; van der Kolk et al. 1991). In particular, those with reported histories of abuse combined with separation and neglect often present with a pattern of tenacious and repetitive engagement in self-destructive activities. It appears that trauma contributes heavily to the initiation of self-mutilating acts and a lack of secure attachments maintains them (van der Kolk and Fisler 1994).

Self-mutilation is related in various ways to a history of trauma. Injuring oneself involves a complex reenactment of earlier and ongoing experiences of abuse wherein the self-mutilator identifies with others who were involved in the abuse. It can be a way to transform an unbearable sense of helplessness and victimization by turning passive into active and becoming one's own perpetrator. By not stopping the behavior, self-mutilators may identify with a passive witness who did not rescue them. They may be expressing their need to punish perpetrators by "using their own skin as a symbol for the offending person's" (Favazza 1989, p. 141) or to punish the vulnerable and helpless part of themselves that allowed the abuse to continue. Self-injury can be a way of ridding oneself of a sense of contamination by the past and perpetrators. For example, in his early thirties, Jay began to recover memories of sexual abuse by his father, which then triggered him to repeatedly pierce his fingers to extract blood in an attempt to purge himself of the presence of his father inside of him. Once he came to terms with his history and had more complete memories, the urge to hurt himself disappeared. In addition, a dynamic that often gets played out by people exposed to chronic abusive situations is a repetitious cycle of pain and relief fueled by a belief that after suffering there is forgiveness and protection (Kwawer 1980).

The various aspects of self-mutilators' histories often get acted out in dramatizations because of incomplete attempts at symbolization of past experiences. The powerful defense of dissociation is often invoked in response to overwhelming trauma and contributes to keeping memories inaccessible to conscious thought. When not yet formulated as episodic memories, past traumatic experiences cannot be remembered as such, spoken about, and processed but rather remain frozen as bodily memories that infuse ongoing pressures to reenact. It makes sure the memories are not forgotten, because one has to remain hypervigilant for future dangers, yet they are never remembered clearly enough to allow processing, mourning, and transformation of the dread of being overwhelmed, retraumatized, and annihilated. According to van der Kolk and Fisler (1994), as long as trauma is experienced and remembered as speechless terror, the body continues to keep score and reacts to related stimuli as a return of the trauma.

An additional factor has to do with the role of early trauma on cognitive development. Maltreated children have been shown to use fewer words to describe internal states, and as they grow up they continue to exhibit difficulty expressing differentiated emotions. These deficits have been held responsible for impaired impulse control. The undifferentiation of affects and the speechless terror that are part of being traumatized interfere with the capacity to put feelings into words, leaving them to be mutely expressed by bodily dysfunction (van der Kolk and Fisler 1994). A pattern remains in which the burden is returned to the body when levels of arousal prove to be unmanagable in the form of fantasies or images (Hibbard 1994). Feelings are acted out with little ability to use intervening symbolic representations that would allow for flexible response strategies. Self-mutilators should be considered to be alexithymic, demonstrating clear deficiencies in their ability to use language effectively to communicate their internal experiences and get help from caring others. Cognitive abilities that could help identify, label, and bind dysphoric affect are absent (Leibenluft et al. 1987). In the case of Sally mentioned previously, one situation that brought on the urge to hurt herself was group sessions in which she was highly stimulated and involved yet did not find a way to express herself verbally, leaving her feeling mute and invisible to others. Self-mutilators with a history of childhood trauma have also been shown to be the least able to use interpersonal resources to help them cope (van der Kolk et al. 1991). Those who experienced prolonged separation from primary caregivers and those who could not remember feeling special or loved by anyone as children were least able to use interpersonal resources to control themselves (van der Kolk and Fisler 1994).

## Implications for Treatment

A key factor in the successful treatment of self-mutilators involves the development of a more sophisticated ability to express things in words, particularly affect and interpersonal needs. In addition to the importance of using words to match and articulate internal experiences, self-mutilators benefit from the growing ability to recount their history in narrative form, in a way that they can take distance from and think of. The process of reconstructing their history is often tumultuous and painful. van der Kolk and Fisler (1994) recommended that clinicians anticipate that painful affects related to interpersonal safety, trust, anger, and emotional needs will be accompanied by dissociative episodes and increased aggression against the self. Therapy will be characterized by phases of acting out and then phases of growing awareness of internal states and their connection to current and past situations. When the mind develops the ability to create symbolic representations of the traumatic and frozen past experiences, there is a taming of terror and "a desomatization of experience." Once patients improve their capacity to endure pain in order to attend to recuperation, much of the work can center on making connections between current stresses and past traumas and clarifying how disruptions in present relationships are a repetition of prior experiences. Words allow distinctions to be made between past helplessness and current ways of coping.

Another aspect of acting out occurs within the treatment, which at times can be pursued only in a later phase, making use of what the therapist and patient reenact as a source of information about the patient and his or her past. For example, by witnessing a patient who is unable to stop abusing him- or herself, the therapist is given an opportunity to experientially understand what it means to be a helpless victim who is unable to stop an abuse. The therapist's task is to metabolize the experience and articulate it to the patient verbally, engaging the patient in an understanding of his or her life history and in a search for new possibilities of relating to others. Allowing oneself to become involved in this dynamic is a way into the patient's internal world through the unfolding of transference–countertransference constellations.

## Interpersonal Approach

Interpersonal theories view shifting and competing configurations of relations between the self and others as the source of most experiences and difficulties that people struggle with. In a similar way, self-mutilation is seen as an act of communication, expressing discouragement, unhappiness, and despair triggered within an interpersonal context. The act is always understood to be an attempt to respond and communicate with others. Early interpersonalists such as Sullivan (1965) and Fromm-Reichman (1960), although not focusing directly on self-injury, were radical in suggesting that suicidal gestures can be the result of a "paralysis of interest in others" (Sullivan 1965, p. 222) or may stand for hostile impulses directed against significant people in the patient's past and current life, or paradoxically against the therapist, rather than being an expression of innate impulses. The focus on interpersonal aspects of behavior is particularly important in the treatment of self-mutilation. According to Favazza (1989), half of the patients studied first mutilated themselves in the presence of someone else, with one-third actually carving words and symbols on their skin in an obvious attempt to communicate. Most cases of self-injury are precipitated by a situation involving a subjective threat of abandonment or rejection by significant others (Simpson 1980). Friedman et al. (1972) noted that in their group of adolescent self-mutilating patients, a constant underlying fear of abandonment characterized transference and other relationships. Suicidal gestures were invariably preceded by circumstances such as rejection by a lover or a mother being hospitalized. Despite the obviousness of such precipitating interpersonal context, self-mutilators often experience their act as inexplicable. Their acts can become increasingly private and secretive over time, characterized by a state of withdrawal and self-engrossment and an unawareness of the impact that their interpersonal environment has on them or that they have on their environment. For example, Matthew, a middle-aged artist, would report violent urges to slash himself that seemed to occur mostly during visits with his parents. Over the course of treatment, his experience of these impulses shifted from sensing them as unexplainable urges coming from within to making the connection that he was responding to covert messages that he be punished and even wished dead by certain family members that were struggling with envy and fury at his separateness. Leibenluft et al. (1987) studied the inner experience of five borderline self-mutilators, most of whom reported a precipitating interpersonal event that triggered a uniform sensitivity to issues of separation, loss and failure. The attack on their self was preceded by intense hurt and rage and wishes to retaliate against the uncaring other.

Interestingly, once the self-injurious act was carried out, the urge to communicate with the other subsided. The act served to replace a more direct form of communication, turning the feelings and actions on the self while withdrawing from the interpersonal reality of the situation; by attacking him- or herself, the mutilator exhibited a regressive slide from object to self.

Self-mutilators experience relationships as highly dangerous; disruptions in present relationships are experienced as a return of past traumas and repetitions of prior abandonment (van der Kolk et al. 1991), dangers that need to be hypervigilantly guarded against. Within the therapeutic relationship, self-mutilation serves various communications that are mostly unconscious, including attempts to coerce others into action or induce a sense of futility and helplessness. Patients may use self-destructive gestures in an attempt to frighten the therapist and destroy the therapeutic collaboration, sensing their therapists' discomfort in the face of their actions (Fromm-Riechman 1960). Repeated self-mutilation within the context of the treatment can be a way of cornering the therapist into a fearful and paralyzed position. Whether intended to be coercive or not, the acts induce a sense of urgency and pressure that may cause the therapist to lose the internal freedom to be able to maintain a calm, curious, and empathic stance toward the patient; the focus instead shifts to paradigms of control and emotional blackmail. The *manipulative* aspects involved in the act include the patient's attempts to force a caring, mothering response from the therapist and to externalize a sense of responsibility for themselves. Therapists often feel compelled to respond with action (i.e., schedule more sessions or phone calls or hospitalize the patient), and become increasingly anxious about their competence and ability to help the patient when the behavior continues. Fromm-Reichman (1960) warned clinicians against becoming controlled by such attempts by assuming the total burden of responsibility for the patient's well-being. Kafka (1969) reported that while working with a female self-mutilator, the "cutting of her arms and legs continued until I experienced fully my inability to save her life. She then seemed to experience more power over her own life, and self-mutilation stopped" (p. 208). The countertransferential responses that self-mutilation evokes (see section on countertransference) make the focus on the manipulative aspects of self-mutilation highly salient and appealing as organizers of the therapist's experience. In this sense it is important for the clinician not to lose sight of the straightforward cry for help inherent in such behavior and of the desperate attempts to make contact with caring others.

## Implications for Treatment

Working from an interpersonal approach, self-mutilation is quickly placed within a relational context. Acts of self-mutilation are repeatedly interpreted as reactions to events in the therapeutic relationship and as attempts to communicate and have an effect on the therapist. The interpersonal approach to treatment advocates a more active interpretive stance than is customary in traditional analytic approaches. Instead of working toward eliminating the therapist's influence by remaining quiet and neutral, the importance of vigilance to disguised references by the patient to the influence of the therapist and the therapeutic relationship are emphasized. The assumption is that when engaging more freely with the patient, the therapist will inevitably enact the role the patient assigns to the therapist without realizing it. The focus is then not on avoiding such enactments but on gradually becoming aware of them and using this awareness in the interpretive work as an invaluable source of data. The work in the transference is guided by the assumption that the patient's experience of the therapist is both governed by schemata associated with early conflicts *and* organized around significant contributions from the therapist in the here and now. The best transference interventions include reference to both. The task of the therapist is to understand and tactfully interpret how the patient is experiencing the relationship, paying particular attention to the contributions of the therapist's own behavior to the experience (Gill and Hoffman 1982). By mutilating themselves, patients are reacting to events in the therapeutic relationship and attempting to communicate and influence it. Thus, if a patient follows a session with an act of self-mutilation, the therapist should inquire into the precipitating events in the session and in the therapist's behaviors that led to the act. The therapist should refrain from rushing to transference interpretations that frame the patient's perceptions in terms of their past. These interventions may be too isolating, burdensome, and beyond the patient's capacity to tolerate and also do not offer the patient the chance to develop in real time a way of negotiating his or her needs in the relationship. One example is the case of Anna, who launched a vicious attack on her skin after a session in which she experienced the therapist as trying to rape her. In pursuing details about her experience, the therapist stayed with events of the session, on one hand establishing a delineation between fantasy and actual events and fostering the development of an as-if quality of transference ("it *felt like* you were raped, however, you were in no way raped") but on the other hand expressing genuine curiosity about the patient's painful experience of being coerced in some way by the therapist's interventions and about the therapist's insensitivity to the patient's cues at the time. Together, they came up with some ideas of how to handle such a situation in the future, including the patient's responsibility to be more vocal in feedback to the therapist when she is feeling pressured. In this case the therapist shied away from interpretations connecting this experience to patient's past sexual abuse, which would have been too overwhelming for the patient.

In their indirect style of communication—that is, injuring themselves in private—patients convey their mistrust of the interpersonal field as an arena in which conflicts can be resolved. The therapeutic relationship is a good practice ground for developing new ways of negotiating needs, disappointments, and conflict with others and of reversing the tendency to mystify interactions and withdraw into a self-contained orbit. The despair, intense neediness, and "emotional blackmail" that can accompany self-mutilation pull for an intense involvement of therapists with their patients. Therapists should guard against the temptation to provide heroic treatment, the end result of which is a reinforcement of the patient's self-destructive potential and a high likelihood of unmanageable countertransference developments as the therapist becomes exhausted and harassed. Therapists should have the internal freedom that comes from being willing to fail in their attempts to save patients of themselves. Therefore, part of the work includes gradually making the patient aware of his or her impact on the therapist and others. It is often helpful for the therapist at the onset of treatment to clearly delineate for the patient how parasuicidal threats or gestures will be handled. Acting out can then be automatically placed in an existing interpersonal context and interpreted as an attack on the treatment and the therapeutic contract. In general, repeated interventions focusing on the interpersonal communications of the behavior lessen the patient's isolation while offering a framework from which it is easier both for the patient and the therapist to understand the nature of chaotic and violent acting out.

It is clear that regardless of theoretic background, many clinicians report a change to occur in the management of SIBs once the issue becomes addressed within the transference, or the relationship. For example, Crabtree (1967) postulated that the early goal of intensive psychotherapy with self-mutilators is the translation of this behavior into an object-oriented dilemma by establishing an interactional transference psychosis. Feldman (1988) concluded that insight itself into the genesis of self-cutting is usually not helpful. In many case reports the turning point in the treatment was when the self-injury was explored as an interpersonal act between patient and therapist. The more traditional psychoanalytic approaches formulate the self-mutilator's development in treatment as a movement from an autistic and autoerotic level of being to an ability to relate interpersonally. Relational approaches understand the behavior to be a regressive slide in which interpersonal issues and communication are mystified, with the therapist consistently not "buying into it" and continuing to address the patient's actions as an interpersonal phenomenon.

## Countertransference and Management

The degree to which clinicians are informed about self-injury and their theoretic approach to treatment will greatly affect the way they respond and handle the pressures of such destructive behaviors. Most schools of psychotherapy require a basic formation and maintenance of a *therapeutic alliance*, which means that both parties work together toward the goal of getting the patient better. In psychodynamic treatment, in which the vicissitudes of the therapeutic relationship are examined more closely and intensified, it is extremely important to keep a thread of the therapeutic alliance going, even when the stormiest, most threatening material is being worked through. SIB poses a powerful threat to this basic premise because it has the potential to put the patient and the therapist at odds with each other: the patient seemingly works to destroy the him- or herself while the therapist becomes isolated in the wish to protect the patient. It is extremely important in such a treatment to find ways to maintain the alliance despite these challenges. These include not losing sight of the self-preservative aspects of such behavior, as described earlier in this chapter, and aligning oneself with the part of the patient that wishes to proceed with their developmental tasks. This vision at times needs to be held on to blindly, with little acknowledgment from the patient.

In the work with self-mutilating patients, intense countertransference issues threaten to overwhelm the treatment and pose challenges for the therapist. These reactions make it difficult for the clinician to remain clear minded and respond to self-mutilation as if to any other clinical matter. Clinicians are often scared away from work with such patients, frequently hesitating to explore, document, and review in depth with their patients the meaning of such acts (Arons 1981). Reflecting a parallel process, a suspicious paucity of literature deals directly with treatment of self-injury. On a systemic level, whole staffs tend to scapegoat self-mutilators. The self-mutilator is immediately singled out by patients, hospital personnel, and therapists (Crabtree 1967). Staff members tend to become split and distanced from the patient and the treating therapist, rationalizing that the patient is being "attention seeking" (Feldman 1988). This may include avoidant and retaliatory behaviors, including refusing to admit such patients (Bennum 1983) and outright aggressive acts; for example, Favazza (1989) reported of a case in which sutures were performed without anesthetic on a self-slashing patient. On the other end of the countertransference reaction spectrum are rescue fantasies and admiration of the willful withstanding of pain. Carr (1977) described a complex reaction among hospital staff members in which the behavior is viewed on one hand as an expression of defiance and attempts are made to control it but viewed on the other hand as honest or pure and evokes respect, envy, and a collusion with the patient. According to Simpson (1980), typical staff responses only encourage further self-mutilation. Simpson goes as far as saying that such behavior "may be far safer and more easily resolved when health professionals are not involved at all" (p. 259). Clearly, staff members working with such patients should be made aware of the typical reactions that tend to emerge when working with self-mutilators and should be encouraged to discuss their reactions openly and frequently. Conflicts among staff members about such patients should be discussed in the open and the patient should not necessarily be shielded from these reactions, the process of making sense of them, or from attempts to reach a resolution (Feldman 1988). A united "front" among staff is very important. Excessive restrictions on these patients are seldomly helpful; they diminish patients' responsibility for their actions and the consequences of those actions and do not foster long-term solutions.

It is important to try to understand the source of such powerful countertransferential reactions. The patient's assaults on him- or herself may cause the therapist to feel abused and victimized because of the disavowal of the alliance and attack on the treatment and the therapist and because of identification with the patient. The inability to stop such behaviors may cause therapists to feel helpless and impotent and can be exacerbated by real or imagined pressures from others, especially in institutional settings. The veiled threat of suicide that is the backdrop to self-injury intensifies such reactions. Clinicians may feel guilt and shame in their inability to stop their patient from destructive acting out, as though this behavior implies something about their own competence as clinicians. This is a complex reaction that probably comprises both the clinician's narcissistic concerns and an experience induced by the patient. The feelings of helplessness, incompetence, shame, and guilt may in turn lead to intense anger, disgust, and contempt as well as devaluation and blaming of the patient. These uncomfortable feelings may lead the clinician to pull away and avoid the patient or refrain from inquiring further into his or her self-destructive behaviors and may evoke an urge to retaliate and behave sadistically toward such patients. This in turn may lead to an exacerbation in the patient's involvement in a reenactment, which perpetuates a vicious circle. Complex issues of control and responsibility are played out in the transference–countertransference constellations with such patients. Therapists often feel blackmailed by their patients; they may come to feel that their behavior is the cause of the self-injury and become gradually constricted in their ability to make interventions. In their wish for the acting out to stop, clinicians unwittingly give the patient a great degree of power. At the same time, by assuming responsibility for the patient's behaviors and developing rescue fantasies, clinicians also assume an inordinate amount of power and may attempt to dominate the patient or release the patient from responsibility for his or her own decisions. The reenacted drama often includes a victim, abuser, unseeing other, and rescuer. Through projective identification, the therapist may find him- or herself feeling and acting as any one of these as well as rapidly alternating among all of them. To a certain extent these feelings are unavoidable; rather than being dreaded, they should be used as a way to gain a deeper understanding of the patient's history and experience while acted on as little as possible.

One of the dangers of such powerful countertransferential reactions is that the degree to which they are uncomfortable for the therapist may lead to an interpretation of the behavior as hostile at the expense of paying sufficient attention to the internal experience of the patient. For example, a therapist experiencing the countertransferential burden of working with a persistent self-mutilator may interpret the meaning of the behavior based on his or her experience of frustration and anger as an indirect expression of the patient's hostility toward him or her. At the same time, the patient's main concern may have been repeated attempts to arrive at a clearer sense of definition of bodily self. Such a discrepancy might lead to a powerful empathic rupture that could easily confuse the patient even more and induce a great deal of shame and guilt. Another source of danger could be powerful wishes to retaliate on the part of the therapist, who may feel abused and held hostage. Therapists often report a dilemma of whether focusing on the mutilations will add a gratifying and reinforcing quality to the behavior and thus may choose to ignore it. They should be aware of the countertransferential motivations for such turning away from the patient's misery and the possible retaliatory motivations behind such choices. Not attending to the disturbing behavior will not free a therapist from the control the patient may be trying to establish. On the contrary, by ignoring the behavior the therapist might easily find him- or herself colluding with the creation of secrets within the therapy and becoming the unseeing other. Self-mutilation should ideally be treated like any other production a patient brings in—with empathic curiosity and within the context of a larger picture while holding on to the frame and boundaries of the treatment.

Therapists working with self-mutilators will benefit from some form of supervision by which they can monitor and explore their reactions. One of the ways to avoid unconscious retaliation governed by unprocessed countertransferential reactions is both to develop sensitivity to the types of reactions that tend to get evoked in the work with such patients and to find ways to communicate to patients the impact they have on others. For example, Crabtree (1967) sensitively distinguished among a feeling that the patient was cutting her apart, empathic pain and desire to help the patient, and a "selfish desire to be a potent therapist" that made her feel hurt, impotent, and angry. Through the course of treatment Crabtree used all of these reactions and gradually communicated them to the patient. Rather than providing the patient with a sadistic weapon or augmenting the patient's sense of guilt, learning about her impact on others served to lessen the patient's masochism. Countertransference reactions are also one of the most valuable tools the clinician has to gain further insight into the patient's experiential world. For example, by observing how objectified and detached he felt during the course of treatment with a self-cutter, Kafka (1969) learned how the patient related to his own body as a "not me" object. He also described how another patient, who did not consider herself fully alive, evoked in him an identificatory stance of "go ahead, slice yourself to ribbons; let's find out if you're alive or not" (p. 210). Kafka understood these reactions to indicate that these patients were stuck in a transitional space between sadistic and masochistic objects, as reflected in the ebb and flow of sadomasochistic transference and countertransference constellations. This transitional space predated the formation of an integrated bodily ego-syntonic membrane.

## Summary of Key Points

1. One of the key points in managing SIBs in psychodynamic treatment is maintaining an empathic stance while engaging in an ongoing, indepth exploration of the meanings of such behaviors to the patient. This includes getting the details of the actual experience, such as seeing the site of the injury; inquiring into precipitating events as well as all thoughts, feelings, and fantasies accompanying the act; and finding out what happened next. The clinician should treat the behavior matter-of-factly, taking the time to collect information rather than presuming motives and meanings, and in that way gradually make the unconscious conscious. Treatment involves an ongoing process of ar-

ticulating into words that which necessitated action and addressing different layers of the experience at different times, starting from the most superficial and accessible. This process of symbolization eventually allows the patient more time to think and freedom to choose rather than feeling compelled to act.

2. Exploration includes developing curiosity and insight into which parts of the self and the other are being attacked. Who is the attacker and who the victim in a given scenario can be complex, multidetermined, and changing; it will be tied to historical relational events and matrixes often revealing sadomasochistic constellations. As the dynamics are worked through, alternative ways of construing and experiencing relationships will become more available.

3. Throughout the work there should be repeated inquiries into the interpersonal context within which the act was carried out. Behaviors will be tied to precipitating events and to communications with significant others in the patient's current life, including communications with the therapist.

4. The therapist should inquire into the transferential context of the act while remaining sensitive to his or her own countertransferential reactions, which may at appropriate times be helpful to share with the patient.

5. An ongoing emphasis should be placed on offering and creatively developing with the patient alternative solutions to the expression and function of the self-injurious acts. Through ego-supporting interventions, patients will develop helpful new distress tolerance skills and an ability to identify and negotiate their own needs. Patients should be encouraged to anticipate distressing situations and make concrete plans about how they wish to cope with these. They can be encouraged to use their environment rather than remain self-contained in their effort to shift states. This includes developing techniques in becoming more willfully immersed in the environment, such as a walk outdoors, music, positive visual experiences, or any external source of interest as well as relating to their own body as a source of soothing experiences and an object to be taken care of, such as by holding an ice cube rather than burning oneself, exercising, or taking a bath. It may also be helpful to train patients in breathing and relaxation techniques (Feldman 1988).

Several concluding remarks end this chapter. When working with self-mutilators, the therapist is continuously searching for an elusive balance between addressing contradictory forces of self-hate and a private sense of grandiosity in the patient. The self-mutilator often holds a combination of an incredibly harsh and punitive attitude toward him- or herself, primitive superego structure, and proneness to drops in self-cohesion and self-worth. These are combined with grandiosity, entitlement, and omnipotent patterns of relatedness governed by a pattern of sadomasochistic control of others through powerful manipulations. The therapist must therefore combine unshaming, guilt-relieving, and ego-supportive interpretations while maintaining a firm stance and solid boundaries. The message can thus be conveyed that self-mutilation is not acceptable but that this does not mean the patient is bad. Work with self-mutilators is often both rich and dicey, with prolonged periods of poor clarity. At times of confusion or when the patient is experiencing an intensely fragile period it can be safest to focus on structure and coping mechanisms rather than content, reserving interpretations for times of greater strength and accessibility.

When treating self-mutilators it is often necessary to transfer much of the focus of the work to the interpersonal domain. This means helping patients become aware of the interpersonal components of their behavior, including self-injury, as attempts to control their own reactions to relational disappointments and anxieties and of the issues of responsibility and control that are inherent in the behavior. Patients should be pushed to develop a reality-based comprehension of the impact that their behaviors have on significant others, including the therapist. Frequently, the therapist's countertransferential reactions may be so powerful, or the patient may be so self-destructive, that it may be urgent to transfer the exploration to the interpersonal arena early into the work before much of the meaning of the behavior is truly understood. When introducing such an approach it is important to familiarize the patient with the impact that his or her behavior has on people, such as the therapist, while maintaining a clear distinction between the behavior's impact (e.g., the helplessness evoked in the therapist), and the patient's intentions.

## References

Arons BS: Self-mutilation: clinical examples and reflections. Am J Psychother 35:550–558, 1981

Bennum I: Depression and hostility in self-mutilation. Suicide and Life Threatening Behavior 13:71–84, 1983

Carr EG: The motivation of self-injurious behavior. Psychiatr Bull 84:800–816, 1977

Cooper AM: The narcissistic-masochistic character, in Masochism: Current Psychoanalytic Perspectives. Edited by Glick RA, Meyers DI. Hillsdale, NJ, Analytic Press, 1988, pp 117–138

Crabtree LH: A psychotherapeutic encounter with a self-mutilating patient. Psychiatry 30:91–100, 1967

Favazza AR: Why patients mutilate themselves. Hospital and Community Psychiatry 40:137–145, 1989

Feldman MD: The challenge of self-mutilation: a review. Compr Psychiatry 29:252–269, 1988

Friedman M, Galsser M, Laufer E, et al: Attempted suicide and self-mutilation in adolescence. Int J Psychoanal 53:179–183, 1972

Fromm-Reichmann F: Principles of Intensive Psychotherapy. Chicago, IL, University of Chicago, 1960, pp 197–200

Gill MM, Hoffman IZ: Analysis of Transference. New York, International Universities, 1982, pp 1–8

Hibbard SK: The mechanisms and meanings of self-cutting. Modern Psychoanalysis 19:45–54, 1994

Kafka JS: The body as transitional object: a psychoanalytic study of a self-mutilating patient, Br J Med Psychol 42:207–212, 1969

Klein M: A contribution to the psychogenesis of manic-depressive states (1935), in Essential Papers on Object Relations. Edited by Buckley P. New York, New York University, 1986, pp 40–70

Kwawer JS: Some interpersonal aspects of self-mutilation in a borderline patient. J Am Acad Psychoanal 8:203–216, 1980

Leibenluft E, Gardner DL, Cowdry RW: The inner experience of the borderline self-mutilator. J Personal Disord 1:317–324, 1987

Rosiello F: The interplay of masochism and narcissism in the treatment of two prostitutes. Contemporary Psychotherapy Review 8:28–43, 1993

Simpson MA: Self-mutilation as indirect self-destructive behavior "nothing to get so cut up about," in Faces of Suicide: Indirect Self-Destructive Behavior. Edited by Farberow NL. New York, McGraw-Hill, 1980, pp 257–283

Stone MH: Incest, Freud's seduction theory and borderline personality. J Am Acad Psychoanal 20:167–181, 1992

Sullivan HS: Personal Psychopathology. New York, Norton and Co., 1965, pp 222–223

van der Kolk BA, Fisler RE: Childhood abuse and neglect and loss of self-regulation. Bull Menninger Clinic 58:145–168, 1994

van der Kolk BA, Perry C, Herman JL: Childhood origins of self-destructive behavior. Am J Psychiatry 148:1665–1671, 1991

# Index

*Page numbers printed in **boldface** type refer to tables or figures.*